THE **FCEM** NOTEBOOK

Revision notes and clinical resource for emergency physicians

Joanna S Rowlinson MB BS MRCP FCEM
Consultant in Emergency Medicine
Queen Alexandra Hospital, Portsmouth
Hampshire, UK

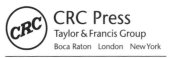

CRC Press
Taylor & Francis Group
Boca Raton   London   New York

CRC Press is an imprint of the
Taylor & Francis Group, an **informa** business

CRC Press
Taylor & Francis Group
6000 Broken Sound Parkway NW, Suite 300
Boca Raton, FL 33487-2742

© 2015 by Taylor & Francis Group, LLC
CRC Press is an imprint of Taylor & Francis Group, an Informa business

No claim to original U.S. Government works

Printed on acid-free paper
Version Date: 20141007

International Standard Book Number-13: 978-1-4822-2483-2 (Paperback)

Library of Congress Cataloging-in-Publication Data

Rowlinson, Joanna, author.
    The FCEM notebook : revision notes and clinical resource for emergency physicians / Joanna Rowlinson.
        p. ; cm.
    Includes bibliographical references and index.
    ISBN 978-1-4822-2483-2 (paperback)
    I. Title.
    [DNLM: 1. Evidence-Based Emergency Medicine--Examination Questions. 2. Test Taking Skills. WB 18.2]

RC86.9
616.02′5076--dc23   2014039281

Visit the Taylor & Francis Web site at
http://www.taylorandfrancis.com

and the CRC Press Web site at
http://www.crcpress.com

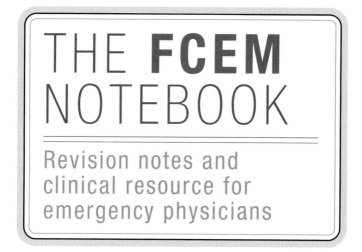

THE **FCEM** NOTEBOOK

Revision notes and
clinical resource for
emergency physicians

To my family

CONTENTS

ENDOCRINOLOGY

ENVIRONMENTAL MEDICINE

GASTROENTEROLOGY

HAEMATOLOGY

INFECTIOUS DISEASES

MEDICOLEGAL

MUSCULOSKELETAL AND INJURY

NEUROLOGY

OBSTETRICS AND GYNAECOLOGY

OPHTHALMOLOGY

PSYCHIATRY

RESPIRATORY

SAFEGUARDING

SPINAL

TOXICOLOGY

PREFACE

The FCEM Notebook is a focused, concise, portable emergency medicine revision resource for FCEM exam candidates and emergency physicians. The examinations for Fellowship of the College of Emergency Medicine (FCEM) demand knowledge, retention and application of a huge breadth of complex clinical information. Extensive personal reading based on the college curriculum is an essential foundation for the exams and multiple literature resources need to be identified and accessed. This book contains short questions related to the FCEM curriculum and succinct answers to allow candidates to revise and test their knowledge as time allows.

Notes below the answers also contain additional material, current relevant national guidelines references and suggested resources for further personal reading that have been selected for their particular relevance to emergency medicine. Space is also available for readers to add their own notes.

This book does not intend to be a direct reproduction of previous FCEM exam questions and the format aims to aid in the retention of knowledge. The question style commonly encountered in the exam is not as direct. The candidate is often required to interpret a stem, establish a diagnosis and then answer further questions. For example, rather than asking directly for the features of Kawasaki disease, an unwell child with fever for six days and red eyes will be described, or rather than asking directly regarding cyanide poisoning, an unconscious patient in a factory fire will be described. Should the initial diagnosis reached make proceeding with the subsequent questions difficult, reconsider the overall diagnosis. Both adult and paediatric EM topics are included within each subsection.

This book is also of relevance and interest to emergency physicians post FCEM refreshing, or helping colleagues preparing for the exams, and also emergency nurse practitioners, trainee nurse consultants, MCEM candidates, foundation years doctors and medical students working within the ever interesting, challenging and enjoyable world of emergency medicine.

Joanna Rowlinson

ABBREVIATIONS

ACE	angiotensin converting enzyme
AF	atrial fibrillation
AIDS	acquired immunodeficiency syndrome
ALS	advanced life support
ALSG	Advanced Life Support Group
ANS	autonomic nervous system
ASOT	antistreptolysin O titer
BMA	British Medical Association
BMI	body mass index
BNF	British National Formulary
BP	blood pressure
bpm	beats per minute
BTS	British Thoracic Society
CCU	coronary care unit
CEM	College of Emergency Medicine
CK	creatinine kinase
CMV	cytomegalovirus
CNS	central nervous system
CO$_2$	carbon dioxide
COPD	chronic obstructive pulmonary disease
CPR	cardiopulmonary resuscitation
CRP	C-reactive protein
CT	computerized tomography scan
CVA	cerebrovascular accident
CVS	cardiovascular system
CXR	chest X-ray
DIC	disseminated intravascular coagulation
DKA	diabetic ketoacidosis
DVLA	Driver and Vehicle Licensing Agency
EBV	Epstein–Barr virus
ECG	electrocardiogram
ED	emergency department
ENT	ear, nose and throat
ESR	erythrocyte sedimentation rate

ET	endotracheal
ETA	estimated time of arrival
FBC	full blood count
FFP	fresh frozen plasma
FVC	forced vital capacity
GCS	Glasgow coma scale
GI	gastrointestinal
GMC	General Medical Council
GP	general practitioner
G&S	group and save
GTN	glyceryl trinitrate
HDU	high dependency unit
HIV	human immunodeficiency virus
HONK	hyperosmolar non-ketotic coma
HPA	Health Protection Agency
Hrs	hours
HSP	Henoch-Schönlein purpura
HUS	haemolytic uraemic syndrome
ICD	implantable cardiac defibrillator
ITP	idiopathic thrombocytopaenia purpura
ITU	intensive therapy unit
IV	intravenous
LBBB	left bundle branch block
LFT	liver function tests
LP	lumbar puncture
LV	left ventricle
mg	milligram
mg/kg	milligrams per kilogram
MI	myocardial infarction
Mins	minutes
mL	millilitre
MRI	magnetic resonance imaging
NG	nasogastric
NICE	National Institute of Health and Clinical Excellence
NSAIDs	non-steroidal anti-inflammatory drugs
OPD	outpatient department
OSCE	objective structured clinical examination
PE	pulmonary embolus
PEFR	peak expiratory flow rate
PICU	paediatric intensive care unit

PIPJ	proximal interphalangeal joint
PPE	personal protective equipment
PR	rectal examination
PTH	parathyroid hormone
RTC	road traffic collision
SIADH	syndrome of inappropriate antidiuretic hormone
SIGN	Scottish Intercollegiate Guidelines Network
SLE	systemic lupus erythematous
TB	tuberculosis
TTP	thrombotic thrombocytopenic purpura
U&E	urea and electrolytes
UK	United Kingdom
UTI	urinary tract infection
UV	ultraviolet
VF	ventricular fibrillation
VT	ventricular tachycardia
VTE	venous thromboembolism
XR	X-ray

CARDIOLOGY

VENTRICULAR TACHYCARDIAS (VT)

VT is defined as a ventricular rhythm of three or more beats at a rate of over 120 bpm.

Can be sustained or non-sustained.

ECG features seen in VT

Capture beats – amidst the AV dissociation an atrial impulse is chance conducted through to the ventricles and produces a narrow QRS followed by an upright T wave (the narrow complex seen briefly thus therefore excludes an SVT with LBBB)

Fusion beats – simultaneous impulses from the atria and ventricles coincide to create a combination complex with a QRS wider than a supraventricular complex but narrower than a ventricular complex

AV dissociation – p-waves seen within ECG not related to QRS complexes (also seen clinically as cannon waves)

Concordance of all complexes

ASSOCIATED STIGMATA OF INFECTIVE ENDOCARDITIS

Osler's nodes (painful raised red lesions on hands and feet)
Janeway lesions (small painless flat red lesions on hands and feet)
Roth's spots (white-centred retinal haemorrhages)
Subungual 'splinter' haemorrhages
Petechiae
Haematuria
Clubbing (now very rare)

READING

Connaughton M, Rivett J. Easily missed? Infective endocarditis. *BMJ*. 2010;341: c6596 (includes Dukes Criteria).

NICE guidelines (CG64). Prophylaxis against infective endocarditis. March 2008.

LONG QT

QT interval is from the beginning of the Q-wave to the end of the T-wave and represents the duration of activation and recovery of the ventricular myocardium.

QT interval is dependent on heart rate, therefore formula is used to calculate the QTc (heart rate corrected QT interval).

QTc = QT length divided by the square root of the RR interval (in seconds).

QTc longer than 0.44 seconds are generally considered abnormal (can be up to 0.46 sec in females).

Causes of prolonged QT interval

Inherited long QT conditions (including Jervell and Lange-Nielsen syndrome and Romano-Ward syndrome)

Drug induced (including erythromycin, tricyclic antidepressants, sotalol, amiodarone)

Hypothyroidism

Hypokalemia

Hypomagnesemia

Hypothermia

Myocarditis

Subarachnoid haemorrhage

READING

Mattu A, Brady WJ, editors. *ECGs for the emergency physician.* Level 1 and level 2. Wiley-Blackwell; 2003; 2008.

ST ELEVATION

Acute pericarditis
Aortic dissection
Benign early repolarization
Cardiac contusion
Hyperkalaemia (later)
LBBB
Myocardial infarction
Normal variant
Paced complexes
Aneurysmal LV
Brugada syndrome
Coronary artery spasm
Hypertrophic cardiomyopathy
LV hypertrophy
Myocarditis
Pulmonary embolus
Raised intracranial pressure
Subarachnoid haemorrhage

READING

Sgarbossa EB et al. *NEJM* 1996.

Diagnosing and confirming death after cardiorespiratory arrest. *Academy of Medical Royal Colleges*. 2008. Available from: http://www.aomrc.org.uk

LOW-VOLTAGE ECG COMPLEXES

Definition
QRS amplitude <5 mm in all limb leads and/or
QRS amplitude <10 mm in all chest leads

Causes
Cardiomyopathy (end stage)
Constrictive pericarditis
COPD (severe)
Hypothyroidism
Myocardial infiltration (e.g. amyloid, sarcoid)
Obesity
Pericardial effusion
Pleural effusion
Pneumothorax
Severe global ischaemic heart disease
Subcutaneous emphysema
(pseudo – gain incorrectly set)

NOTES:

Electrical alternans
Alternating normal and low-voltage ECG complexes
Most commonly seen with pericardial effusion

CAUSES OF PERICARDIAL EFFUSIONS

Aneurysm rupture	Congestive heart failure
Chemotherapy	Dressler's syndrome
Lupus	Malignancy
Nephrotic syndrome	Post cardiac surgery
Radiotherapy	Rheumatoid arthritis
Severe hypothyroidism	Trauma
Tuberculosis	Uraemia
Viral pericarditis (including CMV, HIV)	

CAUSES OF SINUS BRADYCARDIA

Acute MI (especially inferior)

Athletes

Drugs

Hypothermia

Hypothyroidism

Increased vagal tone

Raised intracranial pressure (Cushing syndrome)

Pain

Sino-atrial disease

Sleep

Sleep apnoea

Typhoid

NOTES:

Two double OSCE stations focus on a resuscitation scenario. Resuscitation skills may also feature in other areas of the exam. Ensure in-depth, fluent knowledge of current guidelines. Practice scenarios with your hospital's resuscitation training officers.

READING

http://www.resus.org.uk

http://www.alsg.org/uk

NICE guidelines (TA88). Bradycardia – dual chamber pacemakers. February 2005. Appendix D.

A well patient with no arrhythmias is experiencing
multiple ICD shocks. What is your management?
What does a 'bleeping' ICD indicate?
An ICD patient has received no device shocks but is in
VT with hypotension. What is your management?

IMPLANTABLE CARDIOVERTER DEFIBRILLATORS (ICDs)

Multiple shocks with no arrhythmia:
Presumed sensing errors
Deactivate by placing ring magnet over ICD
Urgent cardiology review, continuous cardiac monitoring and admission to
 CCU required
Device requires urgent interrogation

Patient with ICD experiencing persistent arrhythmias with cardiac compromise:
Presumed ICD failure
Manage as per normal ALS algorithms
Carry out CPR as normal
Externally defibrillate as normal
Administer ALS drug as normal
Device requires urgent interrogation

One or two shocks received, now well, no acute ECG abnormalities and asymptomatic:
Presumed appropriate shock
Inform patient's cardiologist to arrange rapid access OPD review and dis-
 charge home

Unwell patient following shock or more than two shocks received:
Possible new onset of increased frequency of arrhythmia or new onset of
 illness (myocardial ischaemia, electrolyte abnormalities) or coexisting
 drug treatment no longer therapeutic
Full clinical assessment
Urgent cardiology review, continuous cardiac monitoring and admission to
 CCU required

ICD bleeping
Device warning mechanism
Possible imminent device failure, e.g. lead failure or battery failure

Urgent cardiology review, continuous cardiac monitoring and admission to
   CCU required

Device requires urgent interrogation

NOTES:

Patients carry an ICD identification card. Placing a ring magnet over an ICD should not also turn off a pacing function. Avoid external defibrillations directly over ICDs or magnets but do not delay/withhold treatment over concerns of damaging the ICD. CPR can be safely performed with an ICD in situ. Any shocks delivered by the ICD would not be harmful to the person carrying out cardiac compressions. Remember significant psychological sequalae have been recognized in patients following ICD shocks.

READING

ICD deactivation at the end of life: Principles and practice. British Heart Foundation. 2013. Available from: http://www.bhf.org.uk

NICE guidelines (TA95). Arrhythmia – implantable cardioverter defibrillators (ICDs). January 2006.

NICE guidelines (CG109). Transient loss of consciousness. August 2010.

Stevenson WG et al. Clinical assessment and management of patients with implanted cardioverter defibrillators presenting to nonelectrophysiologists. *Circulation* 2004; 110:3866–3869.

HYPOKALAEMIA

ECG changes	Flat or inverted T-waves	U waves
	ST depression	Long QT
	VT/VF/torsades	Prolonged PR
Causes	Diuretics	Hyperaldosteronism
	Intestinal fistulae	Renal artery stenosis
	Liquorice	Laxative misuse
	Insulin treatment	IV salbutamol
Symptoms	Lethargy, weakness, constipation, paralysis, tetany, parasthesia	

NOTES:

Hypercalcaemia ECG findings
  Short QT
  J-waves
  Broad T-waves
  VT/VF when severe

KAWASAKI DISEASE

Fever for more than five days	Sudden onset, swinging, above 40°C, poor response to antipyretics or antibiotics
With four of the following five:	
Lymphadenopathy	Painful, solitary, greater than 1.5 cm
Oral changes	Cracked lips, erythema of lips, strawberry tongue
Rash	Starts in a few days for around 1 week
	Often marked in groin and may peel
	Many forms but not vesicular
Conjunctival injections	Bilateral, non-purulent
Extremity change	Oedema, erythema, periungal desquamation, usually 2–3 weeks post onset

(If proven new coronary artery involvement, only three of above needed.)

Following diagnosis, patients are treated with immunoglobulin and aspirin.

DERMATOLOGY

HENOCH SCEONLEIN PURPURA (HSP)

Widespread small vessel vasculitic process with onset commonly following minor bacterial or viral infection. Most common in 3 to 11 yrs old. Child generally appears well.

Classical findings of:

Palpable purpura (100%)	Traditionally extensor surfaces and buttocks, but can affect other areas
GI symptoms (75%)	Abdominal pain, intussusception, vomiting, haematemesis, PR bleed
Arthralgia (up to 60%)	Especially large joints
Renal (25–60%)	Micro/macroscopic haematuria and proteinuria
Other associations	Testicular pain/swelling/torsion
	Oedematous hands and feet and periorbital
	Seizures, encephalopathy, intracranial haemorrhage/infarct

Admit if

Systemically unwell	Renal failure
Hypertensive	Unclear diagnosis
Increasing proteinuria or haematuria	Poor pain control/unable to mobilize due to arthralgia

Investigations

Clinical diagnosis, investigate to identify complications and exclude other differential diagnoses.

Throat swab	Urine dipstick with MC&S
FBC, coagulation	Protein, albumin
Creatinine	U&E
Calcium	Blood cultures
Blood pressure	Weight and height

Consider abdominal USS for intussusception

Management

Supportive; most have a good prognosis.
Analgesia and rest – paracetamol, NSAIDs (if no renal involvement).

Monitor hydration and nutrition.

Carers can manage at home and with OPD with written advice plan and symptom/urine dip diary if no concerning features.

Prednisolone – can be used if progressing renal involvement/oedema, significant GI features/arthralgia or onset of other significant complications. Discuss with duty paediatrician before starting in the ED.

Describe the presenting features and the skin
rash associated with Lyme disease
How should a tick be removed?

LYME DISEASE
Tick-borne infection caused by *Borrelia burgdorferi*. Most common in southern England in the UK, but also in travellers to Europe and America.

Presentation
Three stages

Stage 1 – Early localized infection
Erythema chronicum migrans rash, flu-like symptoms

Stage 2 – Early disseminated infection (days to weeks)

Cardiac	First degree/complete heart block, myopericarditis
Neurological	Neuroborreliosis, cranial nerve palsies especially unilateral or bilateral 7th, meningitis, encephalitis, lymphocytic meningoradiculoneuritis (Bannwarth syndrome), peripheral mononeuritis
Arthralgia/muscle pain	
Opthalmology	Conjunctivitis, optic neuropathy

Stage 3 – Late persistent infection
Lyme arthritis, encephalomyelitis, acrodermatitis chronica atrophicans (blue-red rash)

Investigations and management
Discuss with dermatologist, infectious disease specialist or immunologist.
Can be diagnosed clinically if history of tick bite and erythema chronicum migrans is present. Alternatively, send serology for *B. burgdorferi* antibodies.
Early localized infection is treated with 14 days oral doxycycline (or oral cefuroxime if pregnant, children under 12, or breastfeeding).
Discuss if other manifestations present.

TICK REMOVAL
Use fine-toothed tweezers to gently pull tick as close to the place of attachment without twisting or crushing. Clean skin with soap, water and antiseptic, and then wash hands. Do not use lighted cigarette ends, match heads, creams, nail varnish or oils. Advise patient to seek medical advice if redness, rash, flu like symptoms

or neurological symptoms develop. Antibiotic prophylaxis following a tick bite is not currently recommended in the UK (discuss if immunocompromised).

Erythema chronicum migrans
Large, painless, circular red, pink or purple rash radiating from tick bite, commonly with central sparing, and well-demarcated edges.

READING

Lyme disease guidelines at Health Protection Agency website: http://www.hpa.org.uk

What descriptors are used in dermatology?
Give five differential diagnoses of a bullous rash
Give the associated causes of Stevens Johnson

DERMATOLOGY DESCRIPTORS

Macule	Flat, nonpalpable lesion <10 mm diameter
Papule	Elevated, palpable lesion <10 mm diameter
Plaque	Palpable lesion elevated or depressed to skin surface >10 mm diameter
Vesicles	Raised, clear, fluid-filled blister <10 mm diameter
Bullae	Raised, clear fluid-filled blister >10 mm diameter
Pustule	Vesicle containing pus
Telangiectasia	Foci of small, permanently dilated superficial blood vessels
Nikolsky sign	Skin separates when lightly rubbed
Köbner phenomenon	Lesions arise in area of previous skin trauma

BULLOUS RASH CAUSES

Contact dermatitis	Dermatitis herpatiformis
Drugs, e.g. barbiturates	Erythema multiforme
Friction blisters/burns	Herpes zoster/shingles
Impetigo	Insect bite
Pemphigoid	Porphyria
Staphylococcal scaled skin syndrome	Toxic epidermal necrolysis

CAUSES OF STEVENS JOHNSON SYNDROME

Infections	herpes virus, EBV, mycoplasma pneumoniae, streptococcus
Drugs	NSAIDs, sulphonamides, salicylates, penicillins, barbiturates

ERYTHEMA NODOSUM

Raised, red, painful lesions (2–8 cm) on shins (sometimes on arms and thighs), often symmetrical. Colour will evolve similar to a bruise over 6–8 weeks.

Causes include

Behçet disease

Drugs (barbiturates, codeine, oral contraceptives, penicillin, salicylates, sulphonamides)

EBV

Leukaemia

Mycoplasma

Rheumatic fever

Streptococcus

Tuberculosis

Crohn disease

Idiopathic

Lymphoma

Pregnancy

Sarcoidosis

Syphilis

Ulcerative colitis

Treat symptomatically with NSAIDs, rest and elevation and investigate for underlying cause (CXR, ESR, CRP, ASOT, throat swab, pregnancy test, FBC and other as per history/examination findings).

ENDOCRINOLOGY

ADDISONIAN CRISIS

Biochemical findings

Hypoglycaemia	Hyponatraemia
Hyperkalaemia	Hypercalcaemia
Raised eosinophils	Increased urea
Low pH	

Precipitants of acute Addisonian crisis

Adrenal haemorrhage	coagulopathy	
	sepsis (Waterhouse-Friderichsen syndrome)	
Abrupt withdrawal of steroid treatment		
Stress with pre-existing Addison disease	surgery	dehydration
	trauma	infection
	pregnancy	burns
	general anaesthetic	
Omission of steroid treatment	vomiting	non-compliance
	iatrogenic	

NOTES:

May co-exist with other endocrinopathies. Addison disease hyperpigmentation can be seen in skin creases, scars, gums and buccal mucosa, skin folds, extensor surfaces.

READING

Wass JAH. How to avoid precipitating an acute adrenal crisis. *BMJ*. 2013;345:e6333.

Give the causes of hypernatraemia, hyponatraemia, hyperchloraemia and hypochloraemia

ELECTROLYTE ABNORMALITIES CAUSES

Hyperchloraemia

diarrhoea
acetazolamide

IV sodium chloride
renal tubular acidosis

Hypochloraemia

vomiting
diuretics

diarrhoea
NG suction

Hypernatraemia

burns

excessive sweating (marathons, heat illness)

vomiting, NG suction
IV hypertonic saline
excessive salt ingestion
nephrogenic diabetes insipidus
Cushing syndrome
HONK

GI fistulae
sodium bicarbonate administration
excessive diuretic or laxative use
central diabetes insipidus

Conn syndrome

Hyponatraemia

Hypervolaemic
    cardiac failure
    nephrotic syndrome
    renal failure

liver failure
inappropriate intravenous therapy

Normovolaemic
    SIADH
    hypothyroidism
    psychogenic polydipsia and other causes of water intoxication

glucocorticoid deficiency
excess intravenous hypotonic fluids

Hypovolaemic
    diuretic therapy
    cerebral salt wasting (subarachnoid haemorrhage, head injury)
    diarrhoea
    burns
    pancreatitis

salt-losing nephropathy
Addison disease

vomiting
sweating

Pseudohyponatraemia

seen with coexisting raised glucose, protein, lipids and mannitol

HYPOGLYCAEMIA IN ADULTS

Use the mnemonic EXPLAIN
Exogenous drugs (alcohol, insulin)
Pituitary insufficiency
Liver failure
Addison disease
Insulinomas (islet cell tumours), infection (malaria, sepsis)
Non-pancreatic tumours (as some release insulin like peptides)

NOTES:

Metformin and glitazones do not usually cause hypoglycaemia. Sulphonylureas can cause hypoglcaemia. Inherited metabolic diseases can present for the first time in adulthood with hypoglycaemia. Inherited metabolic diseases should be considered in patients presenting with hypoglycaemia, metabolic acidosis and high measured ammonia. Emergency treatment regimes for adults and children are available at http://www.bimdg.org.uk and also discuss with an expert.

READING

Joint British Diabetes Societies Guidelines: http://www.diabetologists-abcd.org.uk/JBDS/JBDS.htm

The hospital management of hypoglycaemia in adults with diabetes mellitus.

The management of diabetic ketoacidosis in adults. 2nd edition. Sept 2013.

The management of hyperosmolar hyperglycaemic state (HHS) in adults with diabetes. Aug 2012.

Patient safety and blood glucose measurement: http://www.mhra.gov.uk/home/groups/dts-pcc/documents/publication/con2015464.pdf

What are the features of cerebral oedema with DKA in children?

CEREBRAL OEDEMA IN PAEDIATRIC DKA

Features

Headache, irritability, restless, agitated, incontinence, slowing pulse, rising BP

Reducing GCS, focal neurological signs, abnormal posturing

Papilloedema and convulsions and respiratory arrest (late signs)

Initial approach

Exclude hypoglycaemia

Call for senior help (consultant paediatrician, PICU)

Mannitol 1g/kg (5 mL/kg Mannitol 20% over 20 mins) or 3% hypertonic saline (3–5 mL/kg over 20 mins)

Restrict IV fluids to 2/3 maintenance and replace deficit over 72 rather than 48 hrs

Once stable CT head (to exclude other causes – haemorrhage, infarct, thrombosis)

NOTES:

When Managing DKA treat shock with 5–10 mL/kg 0.9% saline boluses (up to max 30 mL/kg – discuss with consultant if felt to need more). The degree of initial dehydration is commonly overestimated. Do not correct for over 10% estimated dehydration. Do not include urine volume losses in fluid replacement calculations. Fluid rehydration should be delivered evenly over 48 hours.

Antibiotics are not given routinely. Fever is not part of DKA, but DKA can be precipitated by sepsis.

One hour after starting IV fluids start continuous insulin infusion 0.05–0.1 units/kg/hr (dose depending on local consensus). Initial insulin boluses or insulin sliding scales are not used.

Children with DKA die from cerebral oedema, hypokalaemia and aspiration pneumonia.

READING

British Society for Paediatric Endocrinology and Diabetes (BSPED). DKA Guidelines 2009.

ENVIRONMENTAL MEDICINE

**Differentiate between the features of acute
mountain sickness, high altitude cerebral
oedema and pulmonary oedema**

ALTITUDE MEDICINE

Features of acute mountain sickness (AMS)

Recent ascent over 2500 m and headache with any one or more:

GI upset (nausea, vomiting, reduced appetite)

insomnia

fatigue or weakness

dizziness or lightheadedness

Symptoms scored 0–3 depending on severity, higher score = more severe (moderate = score 4).

Treatment – descend or rest. Ibuprofen for headache. Acetazolamide.

Only re-ascend when completely asymptomatic.

Features of high altitude cerebral edema (HACE)

Recent gain in altitude and either:

change in mental state/conscious level and or ataxia in climber with AMS, or

present of both mental state change and ataxia in climber without AMS

Treatment – immediate descent. If unable (e.g. weather) temporize with oxygen, hyperbaric bag, dexamthasone.

Features of high altitude pulmonary edema (HAPE)

Occurs with or without AMS.

Diagnosis:

Symptoms (at least two): breathless at rest, cough (dry or pink frothy sputum), weakness or decreased exercise tolerance, chest tightness (grade mild/moderate/severe)

Signs (at least two): crackles or wheeze, central cyanosis, tachypnoea, tachycardia

Treat – immediate descent, Nifedipine, oxygen, hyperbaric bag

NOTES:

Ref - See Lake Louise Consensus on the Definition and Quantification of Altitude Illness. Acetazolamide acts as respiratory stimulant to improve oxygenation. Side effects of paraesthesia, change in taste, tinnitus and rarely blurred vision.

From *N Engl J Med*, Bartsch et al, Acute high-altitude illnesses, 368, 2294–302. Copyright (2013) Massachusetts Medical Society. Reprinted with permission from Massachusetts Medical Society. Also from *Emerg Med Clin N Am*, 22, Gallagher et al, High-altitude illness, 329–55, Copyright (2004), with permission from Elsevier.

MAJOR INCIDENT

Initial report
Two formats are recognized: METHANE and CHALETS

METHANE	**CHALETS**
Major incident declared/standby	Casualties, number, type and severity
Exact location	Hazards present and potential
Type of incident	Access routes
Hazards at scene, present and potential	Location
Access routes	Emergency services present and required
Number of casualties, type and severity	Type of incident
Emergency services present and required	Safety

Initial approach at major incident scene
CSCATT
   Command and control
   Safety
   Communication
   Assessment
   Triage
   Treatment
   Transport

NOTES:
Patients will be triaged by medical priority to leave scene. Discriminators used for triage sieve are whether able to walk, respiration rate and heart rate.

READING

Course manuals for the ALSG courses MIMMS (major incident medical management and support) and HMIMMS (hospital MIMMS). http://www.alsg.org

HEAT ILLNESS SPECTRUM AND INITIAL TREATMENT APPROACH

Heat rash

Inflamed blocked sweat gland causing limb and trunk itching and red rash.
Treatment – dry skin, remove tight clothes and cool. Flucloxacillin for secondary infection.

Heat oedema

Temporary swelling of hands, ankles and feet.
Treatment – oral rehydration and shelter.

Heat cramps

Painful limb spasms due to electrolyte depletion.
Treatment – rest, stretch, oral rehydration solutions.

Heat syncope

Venous pooling with vasodilatation.
Treatment – rest, shelter, oral rehydration solutions.

Heat exhaustion

Volume and electrolyte depletion.
Headache, lethargy, nausea, vomiting, light headed, dehydration, sweating, tachycardia, tachypnoea, postural hypotension, hypotension, temperature under 40°C.
Treatment – rest, shelter, simple cooling, oral or IV fluid and electrolyte replacement.
Admit with close observation. Recovery over 18–24 hours.

Heat stroke

Failure of thermoregulation.
Temperature >41°C, headache, CNS dysfunction (seizures, reduced GCS, muscle rigidity, ataxia), lack of sweating, tachycardia, hypotension, coagulopathy.
Treatment – resuscitate, rapid cooling to <39°C (cool IV fluids, icepacks to groin, axillae, neck, scalp), sponge with tepid water and fan, may require cooling with peritoneal and gastric lavage or bypass, lorazepam for seizures, catheterize and monitor urine output. ICU admission.
Mortality 10% (multi-organ failure).

NOTES:
Avoid paracetamol as antipyretic. Patients with significant heat stroke may still sweat. Significant heat illness can occur in not excessively hot environments.

Biochemical abnormalities in heat stroke

Acute renal failure	Hyperkalaemia
Metabolic acidosis	Hypocalcaemia
Raised liver transaminases	Respiratory alkalosis
Raised CK	Myoglobinuria
DIC	Hyperglycaemia

DIFFERENTIAL DIAGNOSIS OF HYPERPYREXIA

Amphetamines
CVA
Cocaine
Ecstasy
Heat stroke
Intracranial haemorrhage
Malaria
Malignant hyperthermia
Neuroleptic malignant syndrome
Sepsis
Serotonin syndrome
Thyroid storm

ATMIST mnemonic

A handover tool used by the ambulance service for both trauma and medical presentations.

Age
Time of incident/time onset of symptoms
Mechanism of injury/medical complaint
Injuries/examination findings
Vital **S**igns (pulse rate, BP, saturations, respiration rate, GCS, temperature, BM)
Treatment given
ETA and mode of transport

GASTROENTEROLOGY

Give six medical causes of abdominal pain

What is the Alvarado score?

MEDICAL CAUSES OF ABDOMINAL PAIN

Addison's disease

Henoch Scholein purpura

Hypercalcaemia

Lower lobe pneumonia

Myocardial infarction

Porphyria

Typhoid

DKA

Hereditary angioedema

Lead poisoning

Mesenteric adenitis

Opiate withdrawal

Sickle cell crisis

UTI

ALVARADO SCORE

A clinical scoring system used to aid the diagnosis of appendicitis in adults (max 10 points).

Abdominal pain that migrates to the right iliac fossa (1)

Anorexia (1)

Pain on pressure in the right iliac fossa (2)

Nausea or vomiting (1)

Rebound tenderness (1)

Fever (1)

Leukocytosis (2)

Neutrophilia with left shift (1)

Score

<5 appendicitis unlikely

5–6 possible appendicitis

7–8 probably appendicitis

9–10 very probable acute appendicitis

Reprinted from *Ann Emerg Med*, 15(5), Alvarado A, A Practical score for the early diagnosis of acute appendicitis, 557–64, Copyright (1986), with permission from Elsevier.

PYLORIC STENOSIS
Hypertrophy of the pylorus results in gastric outlet obstruction.

Biochemistry
Hypochloraemic, metabolic alkalosis, hypokalaemic

Presentation
Most commonly between three and six weeks of age
Non-bilious vomiting which progressively worsens and becomes projectile
Initially very hungry then poor feeding and lethargy
Dehydration
Poor weight gain
Visible peristalsis
Palpable hypertrophied pylorus below right costal margin ('palpable olive')
On occasion haematemesis

Investigations
FBC, UEs, blood gas, glucose, split bilirubin, abdominal ultrasound scan

Management
Assess dehydration
Fluid resuscitation boluses 10–20 mL/kg 0.9% normal saline, then maintenance fluids
Correct biochemical abnormalities including potassium replacement
Nil by mouth, NG tube
Theatre for pyloromyotomy (fluid resuscitation is overall priority)

READING

NICE guidelines (CG84). Diarrhoea and vomiting in children. Includes guide to assessing dehydration in children. April 2009.

METABOLIC ALKALOSIS CAUSES

Alkaline dieresis for treatment of salicylate poisoning
Alkali ingestion
Hyperaldosteronism
Massive blood transfusion
Milk-alkali syndrome
Pyloric stenosis, vomiting, NG suction
Sodium bicarbonate ingestion
And other very rare conditions

RESPIRATORY ALKALOSIS CAUSES

Anxiety
Brain stem lesions
Hypoxia
Iatrogenic overventilation
Liver failure
Pain
Psychological
Salicylate overdose

JAUNDICE IN PREGNANCY

Pregnancy-related differentials

HELLP
Hyperemesis gravidarum
Cholestasis of pregnancy
Acute fatty liver of pregnancy

Also consider non-pregnancy-related causes including

Drug-induced hepatitis
Viral hepatitis
Gallstone disease
Autoimmune hepatitis
Wilson disease
Gilbert syndrome

GRADING OF HEPATIC ENCEPHALOPATHY

Grade I   Mild behavioural changes and mild reduced level of consciousness

Grade II   Drowsy but rousable, mild confusion, marked behaviour changes

Grade III   Marked confusion, intermittent agitation, very drowsy

Grade IV   Unresponsive or only responsive to pain

PRIAPISM

Causes

High flow (non-ischaemic)

    Increased arterial blood flow, most commonly from local trauma, not usually painful

    Refer directly to urology

Low flow (ischaemic)

    Reduced venous drainage, painful

    Associated causes

        Sickle cell disease

        Cervical spine trauma

        Drugs (e.g. calcium channel blockers, chlorpromazine, cocaine, marijuana, anti-impotence treatment overuse, anticoagulants)

        Malignancy

Investigations

FBC, blood film, clotting profile, sickle screen

Penile Doppler (to help differentiate between high and low flow priapism if unable with history)

ABG analysis of aspirated cavernosal blood (pH <7.25 suggestive of ischaemic low flow priapism)

Treatment options (low flow)

Ice, gentle walking, opiate analgesia.

Oral terbutaline.

Using local anaesthetic aspirate 20–30 mL cavernosal blood from 10 o'clock or 2 o'clock position.

If not resolved inject phenylephrine following aspiration, liaise with urology for surgical interventions.

Apply dressing to prevent later haematoma.

Simultaneously treat co-existing medical precipitating causes.

NEONATAL BOWEL OBSTRUCTION

Differential diagnosis includes

Colonic atresia

Duodenal atresia

Intussusception

Large or small bowel atresia

Meconium ileus

Necrotizing enterocolitis

Paralytic ilieus associated with
sepsis/electrolyte abnormalities

Pyloric stenosis

Congenital diaphragmatic hernia

Hirschsprung disease

Imperforate anus

Malrotation

Meconium plug

Volvulus

Abdominal XR findings

Can be normal despite significant pathology

Dilated bowel

Perforation

Malrotation of gas shadows

Relatively gasless

'Double bubble' (seen in duodenal atresia, as air in stomach and proximal
duodenum separated by pyloric sphincter)

Target sign/crescent sign (seen in intusussception as two concentric lines or
crescent shaped lucency with a soft tissue mass)

NOTES:

Neonatal bilious vomiting or failure to pass meconium in first 24 hours of birth
require prompt referral to paediatricians and paediatric surgeons for further
investigation. Bilious vomit is green. 98–99% of term neonates should pass meconium within 24 hours of birth and all by 48 hours (can be longer in preterm
infants).

Patients with significant pathology can present non-specifically with mild
vomiting or with severe shock, sepsis or ischaemic bowel. Depending on location of obstruction and stage of presentation abdominal signs can be very subtle. Examine for features of shock/sepsis, reduced bowel signs, pain/guarding,
abdominal wall erythema, abdominal distension, abdominal fullness, PR blood/
patency, vomiting with or without bile (ask to view vomit on clothing). Also
consider and examine for other co-existing syndromic abnormalities (including

cardiac and dysmorphic features [e.g. Down syndrome]). May give history of maternal polyhydramnios.

READING

NICE guidelines (CG37). Routine postnatal care of women and their babies. July 2006.

HAEMATOLOGY

SICKLE CELL CRISIS

Precipitants

Acidosis	
Alcohol	
intoxication	Cold weather
Dehydration	Emotional stress
Hypoxia	Infection
Pregnancy	Sedative drugs

Types of sickle cell crisis

Painful crisis	Acute bone pain/swelling due to bone infarction
Chest crisis	Pain, fever, cough, tachypnoea, pulmonary infarction, hypoxia
Priapism	
Cerebral crisis	Focal neurology, seizures, heamorrhagic or ischaemic stroke, TIAs
Sequestration crisis	Sudden splenic enlargement (most common in children, liver sequestration can occur in adults)
Haemolytic crisis	
Aplastic crisis	Resulting in severe anaemia, often following parvovirus B19 infection
Severe sepsis	Risk due to reduced splenic function (even when taking prophylaxis)

Management approach

Analgesia	Pain score and offer analgesia within 30 minutes to be painfree within 60 minutes, offer IV opiates (avoid pethadine and entonox) with appropriate antiemetics and laxatives
Hydration	With IV fluids and monitor fluid balance
Oxygen	Apply if new hypoxia or saturations <95%
Antibiotics	Treat underlying infections identified
Transfusions	Discuss with haematologist before considering any transfusions
Monitor	BP, oxygen saturations, heart rate, respiratory rate, temperature
Investigations	FBC, blood film, reticulocytes, U&E, LFT, CRP, group and save, MSU

CXR and arterial blood gas if new hypoxia or sats <92% or chest signs or symptoms
Other radiology imaging as per clinical findings

TRANSFUSION COMPLICATIONS

Acute complications of blood transfusion

Acute haemolytic transfusion reaction due to infusion of ABO-incompatible blood

Infusion of blood contaminated with bacteria

Anaphylaxis

Transfusion-related acute lung injury

Transfusion associated circulatory overload

Febrile non-haemolytic transfusion reactions

Urticarial rash

Itching

Hypothermia

ED management of acute transfusion reaction

Stop transfusion.

Assess respiratory rate, oxygen saturation, heart rate, blood pressure, temperature.

Assess for features of anaphylaxis, respiratory distress, cardiac and circulatory failure, urticaria and bleeding.

Move to resuscitation area and give oxygen.

Check patient identification label and compare with the details on the blood product being administered and compatibility label.

Give IV saline (inotropes may be required), catheterize and maintain urine output.

Contact ITU and haematology consultant for immediate advice and support.

Treat DIC, allergic/anaphylactic reactions or fluid overload with the usual therapies.

Inform hospital transfusion department and return blood unit and giving set containing remaining products. Do not use other blood products issued and also return to blood bank.

Take blood for repeat group and crossmatch, clotting profile, renal function, arterial blood gas and save serum. Dip and send urinalysis.

Consider and assess for bacterial contamination (blood product pack discolouration or abnormal smell). Take blood cultures from pack. If bacterial contamination suspected, start broad spectrum antibiotics (as per local neutropaenic sepsis guideline).

NOTES:

Symptoms of acute haemolytic transfusion reactions can be non-specific (pyrexia, flushing, urticaria, myalgia/chest/abdominal/bone pain, tachycardia, hypotension, hypertension, sudden collapse, breathlessness, nausea) and recognition is likely to be late in unconscious patients. Transfusion reactions and related adverse events are reported to MHRA SABRE (serious adverse blood reactions and events) and SHOT (serious hazards of transfusion).

READING

UK Blood Transfusion & Tissue Transplantation Services http://www.transfusion guidelines.org.uk/Index.aspx?Publication=HTM&Section=9&pageid=1143

www.gov.uk never events

PETECHIAE

Causes of petechiae

Disruptions of vascular integrity	Trauma, tourniquets, coughing/vomiting, vasculitis, vitamin C deficiency
Disruptions of haemostasis	Thrombocytopaenia (ITP, bone marrow infiltration, aplastic anaemia, HUS, TTP etc.), anticoagulants
Clotting factor disorders	Haemophilia A, B, von Willebrand disease etc.

Petechiae with fever

Bacteria (e.g. *Neisseria meningitides*, Strep pneumonia, *Haemophilus influenza*)

Viral (e.g. influenza, enterovirus)

Associated disease process – leukaemia, HSP, Kawasaki, lupus

Unknown

Vomiting/coughing illness resulting in head/neck petechiae (SVC distribution)

NOTES:

Petechiae – pinpoint red/purple marks up to 2 mm appearing under the dermis that do not blanch with pressure

Purpura – red/purple marks more than 2 mm appearing under the dermis that do not blanch with pressure

READING

Management of meningococcal disease in children and young people. Meningitis Research Foundation. Available from: http://www.meningitis.org/assets/x/50150

NICE guideline (CG102). Bacterial meningitis and meningococcal septicaemia. June 2010.

INFECTIOUS DISEASES

.

ANTIBIOTIC PROPHYLAXIS FOLLOWING MENINGOCOCCAL MENINGITIS CONTACT

Chemoprophylaxis indicated

Prolonged close contact with the case in a household type setting during the seven days before onset of illness (e.g. pupils in the same dormitory, boy/girlfriends, or university students sharing a kitchen in a hall of residence)

Transient close contact and directly exposed to large particle droplets/secretions from the respiratory tract of a case around the time of admission to hospital (e.g. staff intubating a patient)

Prophylaxis not indicated (unless already identified as close contacts)

Staff and children attending same nursery or crèche

Students/pupils in same school/class/tutor group

Work or school colleagues

Friends

Residents of nursing/residential homes

Kissing on cheek or mouth (would normally bring into close prolonged contact category)

Food or drink sharing or similar low level of salivary contact

Attending the same social function

Travelling in next seat on same plane, train, bus or car

Contact with possible case until investigations make the diagnosis confirmed or probable

Treatment of contacts

Ciprofloxacin one off dose or Rifampacin twice daily for two days, given as soon as possible – following diagnosis of index case

HPA may also advise re vaccinations depending on strains isolated

HPA and public health coordinate contact tracing and treatment

NOTES:

Rifampacin is an enzyme inducer.

READING

Reprinted with permission from Health Protection Agency. Guidance for public health management of meningococcal disease in the UK. 2012. Available from: http://www.hpa.org.uk/webc/HPAweb (File/HPAweb_C/1194947389261)

COMMUNITY-ACQUIRED NEEDLESTICK INJURY

Discard any needles brought to ED into yellow sharps bin (do not send to virology)

Clean wound, wash with soap and water, encourage to bleed but do not squeeze

Check tetanus immunisation status (unlikely to be tetanus prone unless sharp contaminated with soil or manure)

Commence accelerated hepatitis B vaccination as per BNF

If considered to be high risk (source is likely to have blood borne virus, visible blood on needle, needle attached to syringe, deep injection causing bleeding) consult HIV on call to consider HIV PEP (post-exposure practice)

Take blood for baseline serum save for HIV, hepatitis B&C. GP to follow up with HIV, hepatitis B&C bloods at three and six months post injury

If appropriate, advise abstinence or barrier contraception until blood testing complete

Reassure negligible risk of HIV and very low risk of contracting hepatitis B or C through community needlestick injuries

NOTES:

HIV patients attending the ED:

- Avoid stopping/delaying HIV medication. Liquid formulae are often available or HIV on-call consultants can advise on potential adaptations to a patient's regime that can limit the impact, should a temporary gap in treatment appear unavoidable.

- HIV drug interactions can be significant. Refer to the BNF or www.hiv-druginteractions.org.

SEPSIS

SIRS (systemic inflammatory response syndrome) = two or more of:
> Temp >38°C or <36°C
> HR >90
> RR >20 ($PaCO_2$ <4)
> WCC >12 <4, 10% band formation

Sepsis = SIRS due to infection

Severe sepsis = hypotension and end organ changes – lactic acidosis, oliguria, altered GCS

Septic shock = sepsis and hypotension resistant to fluid resuscitation

EARLY GOAL-DIRECTED THERAPY PROTOCOL

Supplemental oxygen +/– intubation and ventilation
Central venous and arterial catheterization
CVP 8–12 (aggressive fluid boluses)
MAP >65 and <90 (vasopressors or dilators)
Haematocrit >30%, central venous oxygen saturation ($ScvO_2$) of >70% (red blood cell transfusions and inotropes)

NOTES:

Surviving sepsis campaign care bundles:

Within three hours:

1. Measure lactate level
2. Obtain blood cultures prior to administration of antibiotics
3. Administer broad spectrum antibiotics
4. Administer 30 mL/kg crystalloid for hypotension or lactate ≥4 mmol/L

Within six hours:

5. Apply vasopressors (for hypotension that does not respond to initial fluid resuscitation) to maintain a mean arterial pressure (MAP) ≥65 mm Hg
6. In the event of persistent arterial hypotension despite volume resuscitation (septic shock) or initial lactate ≥4 mmol/L (36 mg/dL):
   - Measure central venous pressure (CVP), target ≥8 mm Hg
   - Measure central venous oxygen saturation ($ScvO_2$), target ≥70%
7. Remeasure lactate if initial lactate was elevated, target for normalization of lactate

READING

CEM standards – Sepsis. Feb 2013.

Emanuel R et al. Early goal-directed therapy in the treatment of severe sepsis and septic shock. *N Engl J Med.* 2001;345:1368–1377.

Surviving sepsis campaign: http://www.survivingsepsis.org

British Infection Society Guidelines. Fever in returned travellers presenting in the United Kingdom: Recommendations for investigation and initial management. *J Infect.* 2009;59:1–18.

FEVER IN CHILD DISCHARGE ADVICE

Discuss with carer

Seek medical help if child develops any of the following:

Struggling to breathe
Pale, mottled or blue colour
Unable to wake up, drowsy or confused
Neck stiffness
Rash that does not disappear with pressure (explain glass test)
Dark green vomit
A fit
High temperature for five days
Unable to take treatments
Dehydration (dry mouth, sunken eyes, hasn't urinated for more than six hours, sunken fontanelle [soft spot on a baby's head], no tears)

General advice

Prevent dehydration	Offer regular drinks (if breast fed, most appropriate fluid is breast milk)
Clothing	Avoid under- or overdressing and adjust clothing if signs of sweating or shivering
Medicines	Not essential to use paracetamol or ibuprofen to treat fever; use if appears distressed (read dose instructions on the bottle)
Sponging	Discourage, as will not reduce fever
Checking	Check during night
School/nursery	Not to attend if still feverish; notify establishment of the illness

If worried

If you think your child is very unwell call 999 for an ambulance.
You can return to your nearest emergency department at any time without an appointment.
You should also be able to see your own GP or an 'out-of-hours' doctor.
You can get advice at any time from the NHS telephone 111 service.

Collect and review your local ED's discharge advice leaflets. Patient advice is common in the exam.

NICE guidelines (CG047), May 2007 and (CG160), May 2013. Feverish illness in children – Assessment and initial management in children younger than five years.

MEDICOLEGAL

INFORMING THE CORONER

After death in the following circumstances (list is not exhaustive):

No doctor has seen the patient within 14 days before death

Death within 24 hours of admission to hospital

Doubt about cause of death for any reason

Identity of deceased is unknown

Cause of the death is unknown

Death was sudden and unexpected

Suspicious death

Violent (homicide, suicide, accidental) or unnatural death

Related to surgery or anaesthetic

In prison or custody

From an industrial disease or occupational disease or accident

In receipt of an industrial or war pension

By suicide, poisoning or drugs

Result of an abortion

From neglect – hospital, care home, family, self, etc.

Related to medications or drugs (including prescriptions and illicit)

READING

Bereavement: http://www.childbereavement.org.uk/Support/Professionals/Reading and resources

NICE guidelines (CG135). Organ donation for transplantation. December 2011.

Treatment and care towards the end of life: Good practice in decision making. GMC guidance for doctors. July 2010.

NEVER EVENTS

Incidents considered unacceptable and eminently preventable, including the following.

Wrong site surgery

Wrong implant/prosthesis

Retained foreign object post-operation

Wrongly prepared high-risk injectable medication

Maladministration of potassium-containing solutions

Wrong route administration of chemotherapy

Wrong route administration of oral/enteral treatment

Intravenous administration of epidural medication

Maladministration of insulin by health professional resulting in death or severe harm

Overdose of midazolam during conscious sedation following use of high-strength midazolam resulting in death or severe harm

Opioid overdose of an opioid-naïve patient

Inappropriate administration of daily oral methotrexate

Suicide using non-collapsible rails within mental health inpatient premises

Escape of a transferred prisoner from medium or high secure mental health services

Falls from unrestricted windows

Entrapment in bedrails

Transfusion of ABO-incompatible blood components

Transplantation of ABO-incompatible organs as a result of error

Misplaced naso- or orogastric tubes

Wrong gas administered

Failure to monitor and respond to oxygen saturation

Air embolism resulting from intravascular infusion/bolus administration or through haemodialysis circuit

Misidentification of patient, thus administration of the wrong treatment

Severe scalding of patient by water used for washing or bathing

Maternal death due to postpartum haemorrhage after elective caesarean section

READING

http//www.gov.uk/government/uploads/system/uploads/attachment_data/file/142013/Never_events_201213.pdf

CONTROLLED DRUGS (CDs)

The legal requirements and responsibilities regarding the use and handling CDs in the UK include the following.

The Misuse of Drugs Act 1971 controls drugs that are dangerous or harmful. It uses a three-tier system of classification (Classes A, B and C) that correlate with the criminal penalties that will result following illegal activity undertaken or misuse of these drugs.

The Misuse of Drug Regulations 2001 regulates the control and availability of drugs according to therapeutic, legitimate and recognized uses, and potential for misuse. The drugs are classified into five schedules. The regulations were amended following the Shipman Inquiry.

The Controlled Drugs (Supervision of Management and Use) Regulations 2006/2013 details CD handling regulations. Hospitals are responsible for ensuring appropriate systems are in place for CD legislation compliance including stocking, locked storage, storage access, security, ordering and receipt, distribution, prescribing, issuing, destroying, registers, records, accountable officers, monitoring, inspection, auditing, systems for recording, reporting and investigating CD incidents and concerns, maintaining up-to-date standard operating procedures, staff training.

Classification examples (lists are not exhaustive)

Schedule 1	Cannabis, LSD, no recognized medicinal use, specific licence to possess (e.g. research)
Schedule 2	Diamorphine, morphine, pethidine, amphetamine, cocaine
Schedule 3	Barbiturates midazolam, temazepam
Schedule 4	Remaining benzodiazepines, androgenic and anabolic steroids
Schedule 5	Certain controlled drugs (e.g. codeine, morphine) when present in medicinal products of low strengths

Class A	Ecstasy, LSD, heroin, cocaine
Class B	Amphetamines, cannabis, codeine
Class C	Gamma hydroxbutyrate (GHB), ketamine

READING

Read your hospital's CD policy and discuss with your department's pharmacist.

Also read the policy for the management of patients found to be in possession of CDs on arrival to the ED.

MUSCULOSKELETAL AND INJURY

NECROTIZING FASCIITIS
Rapidly spreading infection of the fascia with necrosis.

Clinical features

Significant disproportionate/unexplained pain
Pain beyond margins of erythema
Swelling
Crepitus
Erythema, later purple/dusky skin discolouration
Lethargy
Pyrexia, hypotension, tachycardia
Bullae, later become haemorrhagic
Minor skin changes initially with later rapidly spreading skin changes
Offensive discharge
Skin necrosis
Anaesthesia of affected area
Lack of bleeding from deep tissues

Risk factors/associations

Diabetes	Chronic renal failure
Alcohol excess	Malignancy
Sea swimming	Chronic liver disease
Immunocompromised	IV drug misuse
Insect bites/stings	Minor skin trauma

Post op surgical wounds/invasive procedure/minor procedures

Investigation
Initially a clinical diagnosis, with surgical exploration required to confirm.

Blood cultures, blood gas, clotting screen, U&E, albumin, LFT, CRP, ESR, CK, calcium, wound swabs, cross-match blood
XR and CT may show air in soft tissues and demonstrate extent

Management

Fluid resuscitation
Antibiotics, liaise with microbiology, e.g. benzylpenicillin, clindamycin and metronidazole
Analgesia
Aggressive, prompt extensive surgical debridement
Admit to intensive care unit

Organisms

There are often mixed anaerobic and aerobic bacteria. Organisms include:

Group A streptococcus	*Staphylococcus aureus*
Streptococci	*Clostridium perfringens*
Coliforms	*Proteus*
Pseudomonas	*Klebsiella*

NOTES:

The initial skin wound can be minimal with limited skin findings and the patient appearing well, followed by a rapid deterioration and high mortality rate. Commonly misdiagnosed initially as cellulitis.

**Describe the features of Kanavel sign
and the significance of this sign
Give the causes of a radial nerve palsy**

KANAVEL SIGN

Four components

Finger is held in slight flexion
Fusiform swelling of the finger ('sausage-shaped finger')
Tenderness along the course of the flexor tendon sheath
Pain on passive extension of the finger

Clinical features are found in infection of a flexor tendon sheath in the hand.

Infection usually occurs following a bite or a puncture wound. Early recognition is essential to prevent tendon scarring and loss of function. Patients require IV antibiotics, analgesia and referral for urgent incision and drainage of the flexor tendon sheath.

CAUSES OF RADIAL NERVE PALSY

Compression in axilla 'crutch palsy'
Compression of upper medial humerus – 'Saturday night palsy'
Humeral fracture
Elbow dislocation
Compression at wrist from tight handcuffs or watch strap
Upper arm injections in infants

What are the features of a tetanus-prone wound?
What is the UK tetanus immunization schedule?
Describe the clinical findings in tetanus

TETANUS

Tetanus-prone wounds

Wounds or burns that require surgical intervention that is delayed for more than six hours

Wounds or burns that show a significant degree of devitalized tissue or a puncture-type injury, particularly where there has been contact with soil or manure

Wounds containing foreign bodies

Compound fractures

Wounds or burns in patients who have systemic sepsis

Higher risk

Injecting drug users (tetanus-contaminated illicit drugs, especially through pre-existing skin abscesses)

Heavy contamination with material likely to contain tetanus spores (manure, soil)

Extensive devitalized tissue

UK TETANUS IMMUNIZATION PROGRAMME

Immunization given at two months, three months, four months, four years, 14 years.

CLINICAL FINDINGS IN TETANUS

Hypertonia

Painful muscular contractions, especially face (risus sardonicus), jaw (lock-jaw), back (opisthotonus), neck

Generalized muscle spasms triggered by minimal stimuli (e.g. noise, light, touch)

Autonomic dysfunction

Dysphagia (pharyngeal muscle spasms)

Airway obstruction (laryngeal spasm)

NOTES:

Five doses of tetanus-containing vaccine at appropriate intervals are considered to give long-term protection. Those born in the UK before 1961 may not have been immunized. Immunosuppressed patients who had been fully immunized should be managed as if incompletely immunized. Tetanus toxin causes failure of inhibition of motor reflex response following infection with *Clostridium tetani*.

Spores present in soil or manure, most commonly introduced through puncture wounds, burns and minor wounds. Clusters occur in IV drug misuse population. Mortality 10% to 90%. (Neonatal tetanus is due to infection of the umbilical stump. Clinical findings – inability to suck aged 3–10 days, irritability, poor feeding, rigidity, facial grimacing, spasms when touched.)

READING

The Green Book: http://www.immunisation.dh.gov.uk/green-book-chapters/

COMPARTMENT SYNDROME

Associated causes

Bone fractures	Burns
Cannula extravasation	Crush trauma
Haemorrhage	Intramuscular or intra-arterial injection
Large vessel injury	Over tight casts/dressings
Penetrating trauma	Prolonged lie on limb
Seizure	Snake bites
Tetany	Vigorous exercise

Clinical features

Enhanced pain, pain on passive range of movement, tense swollen limb
Late signs – pallor, paralysis, paraesthesia, reduced pulses

Initial approach

FBC, U&E, CK, coagulation screen, urinalysis (myoglobinuria)
Remove casts/dressings fully
Urgent orthopaedic referral for fasciotomy
Keep limb level with body
Intravenous 0.9% saline
Analgesia
Compartment pressures can be measured

Define the following eponyms

EPONYMS

Bohler angle	Boutonniere deformity
De Quervain	Freiberg disease
Keinbock lunate	Kohler disease
Lisfranc injury	Osgood Schlatter
Severs disease	Simmond test
Terry Thomas sign	Trethowan sign

DESCRIPTIONS

Bohler angle
Angle formed at the crossing of lines drawn from the posterior and anterior aspects of the superior calcaneum on lateral radiographs. Angle less than 20 degrees is seen in calcaneum fractures (but angle can also be normal in a fracture, normal range 20–40 degrees).

Boutonniere deformity
Rupture of central slip of extensor tendon at PIPJ.

De Quervain
Tenosynovitis of extensor pollicis brevis and abductor pollicis longus tendons causing pain over radial styloid. Finkelstein test is positive in De Quervain tenosynovitis (fist is made over thumb and wrist is ulnar-deviated; test is positive if causes pain over radial styloid).

Freiberg disease
Avascular necrosis head of the second metatarsal.

Keinbock lunate
Avascular necrosis of lunate.

Kohler disease
Avascular necrosis of navicular.

Lisfranc injury
Disruption of the tarsometatarsal ligamentous joint complex.

Osgood Schlatter
Pain from tibial attachment of patella tendon.

Severs disease
Inflammation of the calcaneum apophysis.

Simmond test
Test for ruptured Achilles tendon. A positive test if no movement of foot is seen when the calf is squeezed on the affected side (also known as Thompson test).

Terry Thomas sign
Increase in the scapholunate space on AP wrist radiograph indicative of scapholunate dissociation.

Trethowan sign
A line drawn along superior surface of femoral neck should pass through femoral head. Positive sign, indicative of slipped femoral epiphysis, if line is above femoral head.

READING

NICE guidelines (CG124). Hip fracture. June 2011.

Wright M et al. Easily missed? Lisfranc injuries. *BMJ.* 2013;347:31–32.

EPONYMS

Bennett fracture

Clay shoveler's fracture

Gamekeeper's thumb

Jefferson fracture

Maisonneuve fracture

Rolando fracture

Tillaux fracture

Chance fracture

Galeazzi fracture

Holstein–Lewis fracture

Jones fracture

Monteggia fracture

Segond fracture

FINDINGS

Bennett fracture	Intra-articular fracture at the base of first meta-carpal with dislocation/subluxation
Chance fracture	Compression of anterior column of vertebra with distraction of posterior portion of vertabra (hyperflextion injury)
Clay shoveler's fracture	Fracture of spinous process of C6/C7/T1
Galeazzi fracture	Fracture between middle and distal thirds of radius with dislocation of the radial ulnar joint at the wrist
Gamekeeper's thumb	Ulnar collateral ligament injury at the thumb metacarpophalangeal joint (now more common in falls holding a ski-pole – skier's thumb)
Holstein–Lewis fracture	Fracture of distal third of humerus commonly associated with radial nerve injury
Jefferson fracture	Fracture of C1 anterior and posterior arches (following axial load on occiput of head)
Jones fracture	Fracture at the fifth metatarsal metaphyseal-diaphyseal junction
Maisonneuve fracture	Fracture of proximal third of fibula with injury of medial ankle including fracture of medial malleolus, rupture of deltoid ligament/intraosseous membrane/anterior talofibular ligament (external rotation injury)
Monteggia fracture	Fracture of proximal third of ulna with dislocation of the radial head
Rolando fracture	Three-part intra-articular comminuted Y-shaped fracture at base of first metacarpal
Segond fracture	Avulsion fracture seen as a lateral proximal tibia; associated with anterior cruciate tear and menisci injury

| Tillaux fracture | Salter Harris III fracture of the distal anterolateral tibial epiphysis (commonly external rotation injury in 12–15 yr-olds) |

NOTES:

Eponyms should not be used solely to describe a fracture but it can be useful to consider eponymous fractures when initially viewing radiographs. Remember to document whether right/left limb.

READING

Pain management

Clinical standards for emergency departments. *Pain*, Feb 2013.

College of Emergency Medicine. Guidance for the management of pain in adults. June 2010/pain in children May 2010.

Nerve block techniques

Chad S et al. Local anesthetics and peripheral nerve blocks in the emergency department. *Emerg Med Clin N Am.*, 2005;23:477–502.

PARKLAND FORMULA FOR BURNS RESUSCITATION

Total fluid requirement in 24 hours = 4 mL × body surface area (%) × body weight (kg)

>50% given in first 8 hours
>
>50% given in next 16 hours

Use for burns over 20%

Time of initial burn/injury (not the time of writing fluid chart) should be used when prescribing, thus the initial 50% of fluids may, for example, in reality need to be given over six hours following a two-hour pre-hospital extrication

NOTES:

Rule of Nines to estimate the area of adult medium to large burns:

Anterior and posterior arm	9%
Anterior and posterior head	9%
Anterior and posterior leg	18%
Posterior trunk	18%
Anterior trunk	18%
Genitalia	1%
Palmar surface including fingers	1%

OTTAWA RULES

Ankle X-rays indicated if

Bone tenderness distal 6 cm of the posterior edge of the fibula or tip of the lateral malleolus

Bone tenderness distal 6 cm of the posterior edge of the tibia or tip of the medial malleolus

Inability to weight bear both immediately and in the emergency department

Foot X-rays indicated if

Pain in the midfoot and any one of the following

Bone tenderness navicular

Bone tenderness base of fifth metatarsal

Inability to weight bear both immediately and in the emergency department

Reproduced from *BMJ*, Multicentre trial to introduce the Ottowa ankle rules for use of radiography in acute ankle injuries, Stiell G et al, 311, 594–97, copyright (1995) with permission from BMJ Publishing Group Ltd.

READING

Stiell I, Greenberg G, Wells G et al. Prospective validation of a decision rule for the use of radiography in acute knee injuries. *JAMA*. 1996:611–615.

Describe the key features to identify on a child's elbow radiograph

PAEDIATRIC ELBOWS

Specifically look for the following

Anterior humeral line – Drawn along anterior cortex of distal humerus metaphysis and should pass through the middle third of the capitellum

Radiocapitellar line – Drawn through radial neck and should pass through the capitellum

Presence of anterior and/or posterior fat pads

Order elbow epiphyses appear in a child (mnemonic CRITOL)

Capitellum	1 year
Radial head	3 years
Internal (medial) epicondyle	5 years
Trochlea	7 years
Olecranon	9 years
Lateral epicondyle	11 years

NOTES:

The exact age of epiphysis development can vary normally between children, though the order of appearance should always follow as above. Thus, bony changes not present in order should be presumed to be due to a fracture.

Give the complications and contraindications of intra-osseous needle insertion

IO (INTRA-OSSEOUS) NEEDLES

Complications

Compartment syndrome
Fracture
Fat embolus
Haematoma
Infection (osteomyelitis, cellulitis)
Possible growth plate injury

Contraindications

Inability to locate landmarks
Extensive pelvic injury (use upper limb site)
Previous attempts in same limb
Overlying skin infection
Fracture of limb
Vascular injuries on same side
Osteogenesis imperfect

Insertion sites

Tibia (one finger breadth below tibial tuberosity)
Humerus (base of greater tuberosity, palpate for protrusion in humeral head
   with arm internally rotated and adducted)
Distal tibia (proximal to medial malleolus)
Distal femur

NOTES:

Indicated in cardiac arrest or when urgent vascular access is required but not immediately available.

To reduce the risk of late recognition of compartment syndrome avoid bandaging/covering the limb. Monitor limb in comparison with other limb for capillary refill distally, swelling, firmness, colour (pink, pale, blue, white) every 15 minutes. Stop using and remove if clinical concerns and discuss with orthopaedic team re fasciotomy. Cease using IO needles once alternative vascular access has been achieved.

TOXIC SHOCK SYNDROME (TSS) FOLLOWING BURNS IN CHILDREN

Presenting features of TSS in children

Fever >39°C
Rash
Diarrhoea +/– vomiting
Irritability
Lymphopaenia

Treatment approach

Move to resuscitation area
Obtain intravenous access
Send blood and microbiology samples (FBC, U&E, clotting screen, G&S, blood cultures, wound swabs)
Resuscitate and treat hypoperfusion with fluid boluses, normal saline 10 mL/kg and reassess (may need 40–60 mL/kg)
Give intravenous antibiotics, anti-staphylococcal and streptococcal (flucloxacillin and penicillin)
Give FFP 10 mL/kg (repeat if necessary) or immunoglobulin to provide passive immunity against staphylococcal toxic shock syndrome toxin 1 (TSST-1)
Remove dressings, inspect and clean burn wound
Consider catheterization for fluid balance
Manage in paediatric HDU
Review hourly until improving

NOTES:

TSS is a toxin-mediated illness that is challenging to diagnose due to the initial non-specific symptoms that mimic other common childhood illnesses. High mortality up to 50% if untreated, thus early recognition is essential. Currently there is no evidence on methods to prevent.

READING

Young A, Thornton K. Toxic shock syndrome in burns: Diagnosis and management. *Arch Dis Child Educ Pract Ed.* 2007;92:ep97–ep100.

NEUROLOGY

BOTULISM

Toxin produced by *Clostridium botulinum* prevents acetylcholine transmission across the neuromuscular junction.

Presentation

Symmetrical cranial nerve palsies, progressing to symmetrical descending flaccid paralysis, progressing to respiratory arrest

'The Five Ds' – diplopia, dysarthria, dysphonia, dysphagia, descending

Other features include blurred vision, ptosis, facial weakness, dry mouth, postural hypotension, nausea, vomiting, constipation, loss of tendon reflexes, diarrhoea (absence of confusion)

Types

Foodborne (especially home-canned foods)

Wound infection (intravenous drug misusers)

Inhalation (deliberate toxin release)

Iatrogenic (cosmetic use of concentrated toxin)

Intestinal

Management

Antitoxin given early can stop progression of paralysis

Monitor vital capacity and arterial blood gases with intubation as indicated

Inform health protection agency

DIAGNOSES WHICH CAN MIMIC A STROKE

Brain tumour – primary, metastatic

Cerebral abscess

Drug/alcohol intoxication

Hemiplegic migraine

HONK

Hypoglycaemia

Multiple sclerosis

Oculogyric crisis

Peripheral neuropathy

Spinal cord pathology

Subdural/extradural haemorrhage

Todd paralysis

Venous thrombosis

Carbon monoxide poisoning

Cranial nerve palsies

Functional

Hepatic encephalopathy

Hypertensive encephalopathy

Hyponatraemia

Myasthenia gravis

Parkinsonism

Sepsis (neuro or systemic)

Subarachnoid/intracerebral haemorrhage

Syncope

Transient global amnesia

Vertigo

READING

CEM summary of DVLA fitness to drive medical standards. January 2012. Available from http://www.collemergencymed.ac.uk

Current medical guidelines: DVLA guidance for professionals. Available from: http://www.gov.uk/current-medical-guidelines-dvla-guidance-for-professionals

Fernandes PM et al. Strokes. Mimics and chameleons. *Pract Neurol*. 2013;13:21–28.

NICE guidelines (CG68). Stroke – Diagnosis and initial management of acute stroke and transient ischaemic attack (TIA). July 2008.

CEREBELLAR SIGNS (MNEMONIC DANISH)

Dysdiadochokinesia (inability to perform rapid, alternating movements)
Ataxia
Nystagmus
Intention tremor
Staccato/scanning or slurred speech
Hypotonia and heel–shin test inability

Ipsilateral signs

CEREBELLAR SYNDROME CAUSES

Multiple sclerosis
TIA/CVA
Space occupying lesion (primary or secondary tumours, abscess)
Severe hypothyroidism
Thiamine deficiency (including chronic alcohol misuse)
Phenytoin toxicity
Paraneoplastic
Meningo-encephalitis
Heavy metal poisoning
Friedreich ataxia

NOTES:

Causes of CT brain ring enhancing lesions (MAGICAL DR):

Metastasis
Abscess
Glioblastoma multiforme
Infarct
Contusion
AIDS/HIV – toxoplasmosis, TB
Lymphoma in immunocompromised
Demyelinating disease
Radiation necrosis, resolving haematoma

GUILLAIN–BARRÉ SYNDROME (GBS)

Acute inflammatory demyelinating polyradiculoneuropathy

Presenting features

Progressive onset of bilateral, ascending, symmetrical, proximal and distal, limb weakness

Absent deep tendon reflexes

Respiratory failure

Variable paraesthesia and sensory loss

Autonomic dysfunction (hyper/hypotension, arrhythmias, urine retention) can occur

Cranial nerves can be affected (facial weakness, bulbar palsy, opthalmoplegia)

Frequently there is a recent history of respiratory or gastrointestinal infection

Infections associated with GBS

Campylobacter jejuni
Cytomegalovirus
Epstein–Barr virus
HIV
Influenza
Mycoplasma

Other GBS associations

Haematological malignancies
Vaccinations
Post-partum

Investigations

Clinical diagnosis

Vital capacity monitoring (blood gases and oxygen saturation monitoring can be normal and falsely reassuring)

Nerve conduction studies

Cerebrospinal fluid analysis (increase protein in GBS)

MRI brain and spine for alternative diagnoses

Management approach

Plasma exchange, IV immunoglobulins (steroids are ineffective)
Supportive, VTE prophylaxis, physiotherapy

Intubate and ventilate if FVC <15 mL/kg

Mortality up to 10% (from pulmonary emboli, cardiac arrhythmias respiratory failure or sepsis)

NOTES:

Miller–Fisher syndrome is an inflammatory neuropathy causing opthalmoplegia, ataxia, areflexia but no weakness.

MYASTHENIA GRAVIS (MG)

An autoimmune process affecting the neuromuscular junction acetylcholine receptors.

Exacerbation

Pregnancy
Bacterial/viral infections
Post-operative
Emotional stress
Drugs (e.g. propranolol, gentamycin, magnesium)
Omission of drug doses (iatrogenic, unable to swallow)

Clinical findings

Muscle fatigue and weakness on exercise, improves with rest (e.g. unable to sustain upward gaze or complete counting to 50)
Ocular muscle weakness ptosis, diploplia (most common)
Head drop (neck muscle weakness)
Limb weakness (proximal > distal)
Slurred speech
Dysphagia
Respiratory muscle weakness leading to respiratory failure
(Normal reflexes, tone and sensation, no muscle wasting)

Management approach

Monitor vital capacity and arterial blood gases.
Refer to neurology and ITU for consideration of immunoglobulin, plasma-pheresis, immunosuppression.

NOTES:

Myasthenic crisis can be difficult to differentiate between cholinergic crisis (i.e. overuse of anticholinergic medication – pyridostigmine). Cholinergic crisis is associated with sweating, miosis, salivation, fasciculations.

Eaton–Lambert syndrome – Autoimmune process against calcium channels on motor nerves resulting in lack of acetylcholine. Most commonly a paraneoplastic syndrome associated with small cell lung cancer. Similar presentation to MG but limb weakness is predominant feature. Investigate for underlying malignancy.

READING

Spillane J et al. Myasthenia gravis, easily missed? *BMJ.* 2012;345:e8497.

FITTING CHILD

Note time and start clock.
Assess and protect airway and give high flow oxygen.
Check blood glucose level.

1. Five minutes after convulsion started	Administer benzodiazepine (IV route first choice)
	Rectal diazepam 0.5 mg/kg (max 20 mg)
	Buccal Midazolam 0.5 mg/kg (max 10 mg)
	Lorazepam 0.1 mg/kg IV/IO (max 4 mg) or
	Diazepam IV
2. Seizure for further 10 mins post step 1	Administer second dose of benzodiazedpine
	Call for senior help
	Start to prepare phenytoin
3. Seizure for further 10 mins post step 2	Give phenytoin 20 mg/kg IV/IO over 20 mins
	If already on phenytoin give phenobarbitone 20 mg/kg IV/IO over 5–10 minutes
4. Seizure for further 20 mins post step 3	RSI with thiopentone 4 mg/kg IV/IO

NOTES:

Carers may carry a personal emergency status epilepticus treatment plan.

Give the features in history and examination
which would be important to elicit in a six-year-old
presenting following a first fit

PAEDIATRIC FIRST FIT

Important history findings

Seizure lasting more than 10 minutes
Required more than one dose of benzodiazepine
Focal seizure
Drugs, alcohol or toxins
Head injury
Pre-existing neurological condition
Pre-existing syndrome diagnosis
Developmental delay or regression
Bleeding disorder
Immunosuppression

Important examination findings

Febrile	Appears unwell
GCS not returned to 15	Focal neurology
Signs of meningism	Signs of raised intracranial pressure
Abnormal observations	Abnormal head circumference
Dysmorphic features	Abnormal cardiac examination

Fitting child minimum investigations include BM, temperature, ECG, MSU (and pregnancy test in older children). Fully undress and examine.

OBSTETRICS AND GYNAECOLOGY

What is your initial approach on identification
of umbilical cord prolapse?
Describe the APGAR score

UMBILICAL CORD PROLAPSED

ED approach

Knees to chest.

Insert size 16 Foley catheter into bladder. Fill with 500 mL normal saline (or until presence of distended bladder above pubis). Inflate balloon and clamp catheter.

Urgent obstetric assessment re presence of cord pulsation, fetal heart beat, fetal movements, and transfer to theatre for caesarean section.

APGAR SCORE

Numeric evaluation of condition at birth. Score at one minute and five minutes post birth.

Colour	Blue/pale (0)
	Pink body, blue limbs (1)
	Pink (2)
Heart rate	Absent (0)
	<100 (1)
	>100 (2)
Reflex irritability	No response to stimulus (0)
	Grimace (1)
	Strong cough/sneeze/cry (2)
Tone	Limp (0)
	Flexed limbs with minimal movement (1)
	Active movement (2)
Breathing	Absent (0)
	Irregular gasping/slow (1)
	Normal/crying (2)
Score	7–10 = normal

Mnemonic APGAR

Appearance, **P**ulse, **G**rimace, **A**ctivity, **R**espiration

PRE-ECLAMPSIA AND ECLAMPSIA

Symptoms and signs

Headache
Visual disturbances (flashing, floaters)
Vomiting
Epigastric pain
Nondependent (especially facial) or pulmonary oedema
Right upper quandrant pain
Recent hypertension >160/110 with proteinuria >1 g in 24 hr
Hypereflexia with clonus

Management approach imminent eclampsia or eclampsia

Initial approach	Left tilt, assess and protect airway, apply oxygen, ventilate as required, assess pulse and BP, IV access
Call for help	Senior obstetric anaesthetist, obstetrician, neonatologist, midwife, emergency physician, intensive care, haematologist
Seizures	Magnesium IV load 4 g over 10–20 min followed by 1 g/hr infusion
Ongoing seizures	Further $MgSO_4$ (2 g under 70 kg, 4 g over 70 kg) over 5–10 min
	Diazepam 10 mL IV or IV thiopentone 3–5 mg/kg paralyze, intubate and ventilate
Hypertension	Treat if systolic >170 or diastolic >110 or MAP >125
	Hydralazine, labetolol
Deliver	Once mother stabilized, deliver baby; fetal heart rate and CTG monitoring
Investigations	FBC, platelets, U&E, LFT, urate, clotting, group and save, urine
Fluid balance	Avoid iatrogenic fluid overload

NOTES:

Hypermagnasaemia

Review magnesium levels and stop infusion if:

- Urine output <100 mL in 4 hr
- Patella reflexes absent
- Respiratory rate <16/min
- Oxygen saturations <90%

Symptoms

- Feeling warm
- Flushing
- Double vision
- Slurred speech
- Loss of tendon reflexes
- Respiratory depression then arrest
- Cardiac arrest

Management

- 10% calcium gluconate 10 mL over 10 min

HELLP

Can occur with severe pre-eclampsia:

Haemolysis
Elevated Liver enzymes
Low Platelets

READING

NICE guidelines (CG107). Hypertension in pregnancy. August 2010.

SHOULDER DYSTOCIA

The following mnemonic can help in shoulder dystocia. The order of manoeuvres is not essential. Mnemonic HELPERR:

Call for **H**elp (obstetric consultant, obstetric anaesthetist, midwife, neonatology).

Evaluate for episiotomy (may not help resolve the shoulder dystocia in itself but allows more space to perform internal manoeuvres and reduces significant vaginal lacerations).

Legs into McRobert's manoeuvre. Flex, abduct and rotate both thighs outwards (straightens sacrum and causes cephalic rotation of the pelvis to help free an impacted shoulder).

Pressure (suprapubic).

Enter for rotatory manoeuvres.

Remove the posterior arm.

Roll (Gaskin manoeuvre; move to an all-fours position with the back arched).

Most cases of shoulder dystocia are unpredictable.

Complications of shoulder dystocia include cerebral hypoxia, cerebral palsy, fracture of clavicle, fracture of humerus, brachial plexus injury, post-partum haemorrhage, vaginal and perianal lacerations, uterine rupture.

CAUSES OF POST-PARTUM HAEMORRHAGE

Tone	Reduced uterine tone
Tissue	Retained placenta
	Retained products
	Placenta praevia
	Uterine inversion
Tear	Genital tract trauma
	Uterine rupture
Thrombin	Coagulopathy

READING

MOET course manual ALSG (Managing Obstetric Emergencies and Trauma).

OPHTHALMOLOGY

RETROBULBAR HAEMORRHAGE

Clinical findings

Reduced visual acuity   Raised intraocular pressure
Proptosis   Afferent pupilliary defect
Reduced eye range of movement   Painful eye/movement
Subconjunctival haemorrhage   Pale retina

Causes

Trauma   Post-operative
Spontaneous   Coagulopathy

Management

Lateral canthotomy
Medical options include mannitol, acetazolamide, dexamethasone but lateral canthotomy should be first line
Sight threatening emergency

NOTES:

YouTube has several examples of how to perform a lateral canthotomy.

PAPILLOEDEMA

Differential diagnosis

Raised intracranial pressure (tumour, hydrocephalus, abscess, subdural haematoma, etc.)

Venous thrombosis

Benign (idiopathic) intracranial hypertension

Central retinal vein thrombosis

Meningitis

Grade 4 hypertensive retinopathy

Drug toxicity (e.g. tetracycline, lead, vitamin A)

Hypoparathyroidism

Hypercapnoea

CENTRAL RETINAL ARTERY OCCLUSION

Clinical findings

Sudden, painless, striking, unilateral vision loss (finger counting acuity
occurring in seconds)
Pale retina with cherry red spot
Afferent pupilliary defect

Causes

Hypertension
Diabetes
Atherosclerosis
Sickle cell disease
Atrial fibrillation
Embolism
Endocarditis
Patent foramen ovale
Intravenous drug misuse
Arteritis/vasculitidies
Migraine
Hypercoagulopathies
Polycythaemia
Arterial spasm
Dissection

NOTES:

Avoid giving answers that are already inferred in the question (e.g. if the stem
has stated the patient has atrial fibrillation and asks for associations with retinal
artery occlusion, points would not be awarded for writing atrial fibrillation).

READING

Beatty S, Au Eong KG. Acute occlusion of the retinal arteries: Current concepts
and recent advances in diagnosis and management. *EMJ.* 2000;**17**:324–329.

Khaw PT et al. *ABC of Eyes.* BMJ Books.

**What are the fundoscopy findings in
central retinal vein occlusion?
Which conditions are associated with
central retinal vein occlusion?**

RETINAL VEIN OCCLUSION

Sudden unilateral painless blurring/reduced/loss of vision
Branch (more common) or central retinal vein occlusion

Fundoscopy ('stormy sunset')

Widespread flame haemorrhages
Optic disc swelling
Cotton-wool spots
Dilated retinal veins
Afferent pupillary defect

Associations

Diabetes	Glaucoma
Hypertension	Hyperviscosity syndromes (myeloma, leukaemias)
Hyperlipidaemia	Obesity
Sarcoid	Smoking
Thrombophilias	Vasculitis

Investigations

Visual acuity	BP
ECG	BM
Cholesterol and lipids	FBC and blood film
ESR	

Others as indicated by history (plasma protein electrophoresis, thrombo-
philia screening, etc.)

NOTES:

History points for loss of vision. Enquire whether sudden, one or both eyes, painful, redness, transient or persistent, trauma, headache, temporal pain, other neurological signs, medical history (AF, TIA, etc.), all of vision versus hemianopia/
quantrantanopia/central, distorted vision, flashers, floaters, toxins (methanol).

What is Seidel's test?

EYE TRAUMA

Seidel's test: uses fluorescein to identify a corneal wound causing an aqueous humour leak. Fluorescein will appear to dilute in a stream across the surface of the cornea (a negative test does not exclude a corneal wound).

Following blunt or penetrating trauma document and examination for

Bone pain
Diploplia
Eye movements
Globe intact
Intra-ocular haemorrhage
Iris irregularity
Periorbital bruising
Pupilliary abnormalities –
reactive/irregular/shape
Retinal haemorrhage/detachment
Subconjunctival haemorrhage
Visual acuity and fields

Corneal abrasions/clouding
Eye emphysema
Eyelid wounds
Hyphaema
Infra orbital paraesthesia
Lens dislocation
Proptosis

Red reflex
Soft tissue swelling
Traumatic mydriasis

NOTES:

The 'black eyebrow sign' is commonly missed on facial X-rays. A lucent (blacker) area is seen by the superior orbital rim on the affected sign which mimics an eyebrow. Indicates free air/intraorbital emphysema following an orbital blow-out fracture.

**A patient presents with painful eyes
following a day walking in snow.
What is the likely diagnosis?**

PHOTOKERATITIS

Eye exposure to ultraviolet light damages the corneal epithelium.

History of UV exposure without wearing appropriate eye protection – examples:

> Welding
>
> Sun reflection during snow/ice/water activities
>
> Sunbed use
>
> Viewing direct sunlight

Symptoms onset 4 to 12 hours after exposure:

> Pain
>
> Watering eyes
>
> Foreign body sensation
>
> Photophobia
>
> Reduced visual acuity (mild)
>
> Eye erythema
>
> Periorbital skin redness

Both eyes should be symptomatic (consider alternative diagnosis if unilateral).

Fluorescein staining shows diffuse punctuate uptake.

Management

Oral analgesia (NSAIDs), sunglasses, advise to not use contact lenses

Reassure symptoms should improve over 1–2 days

Re-present if symptoms worsen or do not resolve

Give advice regarding UV light and appropriate eye protection

PSYCHIATRY

DIFFERENTIAL DIAGNOSIS OF PSYCHOSIS

Recreational drugs (acute use, chronic use or abrupt withdrawal)

Cocaine	Amphetamines
Alcohol	Cannabis
Hallucinogenics	

Drugs

Corticosteroids	Mefloquine
Propranolol	Levodopa

Electrolyte disturbance

Hyponatraemia

Hyper/hypocalaemia

Hypoglycemia

Endocrine

Hyper/hypothyroidism

Cushing disease

Infective

Sepsis	Cerebral malaria
HIV	Encephalitis

Metabolic

Hepatic encephalopathy	Acute intermittent porphyria
Wilson disease	Niacin deficiency
Thiamine deficiency	B12 deficiency
Inherited metabolic disorder	

Neurological

Dementia	Acute/chronic head injury
Cerebral tumours	Multiple sclerosis
CVA	Migraine
Huntington disease	Following seizure (post ictal)

Other

Post-partum	SLE
Heavy metal poisoning	Hypoxia
Paraneoplastic	

NOTES:

The most common cause is drug-induced from recreational, prescription or over-the-counter drugs. An organic cause should be considered in the ED prior to attributing to a primary psychotic disorder. An organic cause of psychosis can co-exist with a psychiatric diagnosis.

ASSESSING CAPACITY

Lack of capacity requires demonstration of both

Impairment of or disturbance in functioning of mind or brain, and
Inability to do any of the following (mnemonic CURB):

Communicate decision
Understand information given
Retain the information to use for a decision
Balance: Weigh up the treatment options/information

Mental Capacity Act principles

Assume capacity
Take all practical steps to enable a person to make own decisions
Help people who have capacity
An unwise decision does not equal a lack of capacity
Decisions for people without capacity should be in their best interests
Decisions should be least restrictive as possible

NOTES:

Mental capacity assessments are decision specific.

READING

The Mental Capacity Act: http://www.legislation.gov.uk

Capacity assessment in children – GMC guidance 0–18 years: guidance for all doctors.

MENTAL HEALTH ACT

Section 2	Admission for assessment up to 28 days
Section 3	Admission for treatment up to 6 months
Section 5(2)	Compulsory detention of patient already receiving inpatient treatment for up to 72 hours by a doctor
Section 136	Police officer detains in a public place to a place of safety

RESPIRATORY

SVCO (SUPERIOR VENA CAVA OBSTRUCTION)

Reduction of venous return through the SVC to the right atrium due to tumour invasion of vessel wall, blood clot obstructing the lumen or external pressure.

Clinical features

Fixed dilated neck, anterior chest wall and arm veins
Face, neck, upper chest, arm oedema
Plethoric or cyanosed face
Conjunctival injection
Hoarseness, stridor
Dysphagia
Headaches, heady fullness
Breathlessness
Chest pain
Facial flushing, congestion and stridor may worsen on raising both arms
    (Pemberton sign)

Causes

Primary lung cancer (most common cause)
Retrosternal tumours (including lymphoma, thymoma)
SVC catheter complications (thrombosis)
Retrosternal goitre
Mediastinal lymphadenopathy (lymphoma)
Aortic aneurysm
Mediastinitis

NOTES:

An oncological/surgical emergency. Image for underlying cause with CXR, CT/MRI, venogram. Nurse sitting up.

Depending on underlying cause treatment includes dexamethasone, chemotherapy, radiotherapy, antiocoagulation, stents, surgical resection.

PNEUMOMEDIASTINUM

Causes

Asthma
Boerhaave syndrome (oesophageal rupture following vomiting)
Blunt/penetrating chest trauma
Diving
Iatrogenic following endobronchial or oesophageal procedure
Illicit drug inhalation
Mechanical ventilation
Perforated bowel
Pnemothorax
Spontaneous

(Most common listed; literature lists many other case associations)

Hamman sign can be found with pneumomediastinum – crunching sound heard synchronous with the heartbeat

NOTES:

Causes of life threatening chest injuries (ATOM FC):

Airway obstruction
Tension pneumothorax
Open pneumothorax
Massive haemothorax
Flail chest
Cardiac tamponad

READING

Wise D et al. Emergency thoracotomy: "how to do it." *Emerg Med J.* 2005;22:22–24.

PREDICTING DIFFICULT AIRWAYS

LEMON – predicts difficult laryngoscopy and intubation if score 5 or more

Look	Face trauma, big incisors, beard, moustache, big tongue (1 point each)
Evaluate (3-3-2 rule)	Inter-incisor distance <3 finger breadths
	Hyoid–mental distance <3 finger breadths
	Thyroid–floor of mouth <2 finger breadths
	(1 point each)
Mallampati	Score 3 or more (1 point)
Obstruction	Tumours, epiglottitis etc.
Neck mobility	Limited, e.g. rheumatoid arthritis

MOANS – predicts difficult bag-valve-mask

Mask seal	Likely inadequate, e.g. trauma, beard
Obesity	BMI >26
Age	55 years old +
No teeth	
Stiff ventilation	Late pregnancy, ARDS, COPD, asthma

SHORT – predicts difficult cricothyroidotomy

Surgery	Prior neck surgery
Haematoma	Significant neck haematoma
Obesity	BMI >26
Radiation	Prior neck radiation
Tumour	Neck tumours

Give the causes of the following capnography
traces in an intubated patient:
sudden loss of trace, gradually increasing trace,
slanted expiratory trace, gradually falling size

CAPNOGRAPHY TRACES

Straight line/sudden loss of trace

Cardiac arrest
Capnograph sampling tubing blockage
Disconnected capnograph
Dislodged ET tube
Lung blockage (e.g. severe bronchospasm)
Respiratory arrest/no breaths bagged
Obstruction of airway (e.g. foreign body, tracheal tube obstruction)
Ventilator faulty

Gradually increasing size

Inadequate ventilation (hypoventilation)
Increased CO_2 production (e.g. malignant hyperpyrexia)
Pain
Respiratory depressant drugs
Shivering

Slanted expiratory trace

Incomplete exhalation
Partial obstruction of airway (e.g. tracheal tube secretions, kinking)
Partial obstruction of lungs (e.g. bronchospasm, COPD, mucous plugging)
Poor sampling technique

Gradually falling size

Cardiopulmonary arrest
Dead space ventilation
Hyperventilating
Hypothermia
Massive blood loss
PE
Sudden hypotension

Other traces

Saw-like mini waves/ripple	cardiac oscillations
Stepwise gradually rising baseline	re-breathing
Small dips along plateau phase	relaxation notches

NOTES:

Oesophageal intubation can cause:

Flat line
Abnormally shaped capnograms with a gradually falling trace
Small irregular humps

DOPES mnemonic – differential for loss of capnography/desaturation in an intubated patient

Displacement	Tube migration above cord, oesophageal intubation, right main bronchus intubation
Obstruction	Blocked tube (mechanical kink/bitten, secretions, bronchospasm)
Pneumothorax	Decompress if clinical signs
Equipment	Disconnected from oxygen/ventilator, ventilator failure, oxygen supply failure
Sensitivity and Stomach	Impending anaphylaxis (e.g. contract media, antibiotic), respiratory compromised due to gastric distension (especially in children)

ECHOCARDIOGRAPHY FINDINGS IN SIGNIFICANT PULMONARY EMBOLISM (PE)

Right ventricle dilatation
Right ventricle diffusely hypokinetic
Right atrial dilatation
Septal flattening/paradoximal movement
Pulmonary artery dilatation
Tricuspid regurgitation
Dilated non-collapsing inferior vena cava
Elevated pulmonary pressures

READING

NICE guidelines (CG144). Venous thromboembolic diseases. June 2012.

Wells PS et al. Evaluation of D-dimer in the diagnosis of suspected deep-vein thrombosis. *N Engl J Med.* 2003;349:1227–1235.

CAUSES OF CAVITATING LUNG LESIONS

Abscess	Brochogenic carcinoma
Fungal infection	Hydatid cyst
Lung infarction	Tuberculosis
Wegener granulomatosis	

CAUSES OF LUNG ABSCESSES

Actinomycosis	Amoebic abscess
Aspergillus	*Klebsiella*
Staph aureus	Tuberculosis

READING

Non-invasive ventilation in chronic obstructive pulmonary disease. Management of acute type 2 respiratory failure. RCP/BTS guidelines. October 2008.

PNEUMONIA

CURB65 score, used to assess severity of community acquired pneumonia. Score 1 point for each.

New **C**onfusion
Urea >7 mmol/L
Respiratory rate ≥30/min
Blood pressure <90 systolic or ≤60 diastolic
Age ≥**65**

    0 = Low severity, likely suitable for home treatment
    1–2 = Moderate severity
    3–4 = High severity and risk of death. ICU involvement recommended

NOTES:

Clinical judgement, the patient's social circumstances and the presence of other coexisting pathology should be considered along with the CURB65 score when assessing severity and deciding location for treatment.

Reproduced from *BTS Guidelines for the Management of Community Acquired Pneumonia in Adults*, copyright (2009) with permission from BMJ Publishing Group Ltd.

What is the differential diagnosis of new onset stridor in a three-year-old?
Suggest features to differentiate between causes of stridor
Describe the UK childhood immunization schedule

PAEDIATRIC STRIDOR DIFFERENTIAL DIAGNOSES

Croup	Inspiratory stridor, barking cough, mild fever, possible preceding coryza, night presentation
Inhaled foreign body	Sudden onset in previously well child, afebrile, history of choking/gagging
Epiglotittis	Systemically unwell, fever >38.5°C, soft stridor, limited/no cough, drooling, rapid onset, unimmunized
Allergic angioedema	Periorbital oedema, lip swelling, urticarial rash, pruritis, shock
Bacterial tracheitis	Moderate to high fever, drooling
Abscess (tonsillar or retropharyngeal)	High fever, dysphagia/painful swallow, neck hyperextension/painful range of movement/swelling, trismus, smoke/chemical irritation, detailed pre-hospital history, similar symptoms in family

UK CHILDHOOD IMMUNIZATION SCHEDULE

Two months	Diphtheria, tetanus, pertussis, polio, haemophilus influenza type b, pnemococcal, rotavirus
Three months	Diphtheria, tetanus, pertussis, polio, haemophilus influenza type b, meningococcal group C, rotavirus
Four months	Diphtheria, tetanus, pertussis, polio, haemophilus influenza type b, pnemococcal
12 to 13 months	Haemophilus influenza type b, meningitis group C, pnemococcal, measles, mumps, rubella
Three years four months	Diphtheria, tetanus, pertussis, polio, measles, mumps, rubella
12 to 13 years	Human papillomavirus (girls)
14 years	Tetanus, diphtheria, polio, meningitis C

CROUP

Assessing croup severity

Westley croup score (mnemonic SCARE)

Stridor   0 = none, 1 = with agitation, 2 = at rest

Cyanosis   0 = none, 4 = with agitation, 5 = at rest

Alertness   0 = normal, 5 = disorientated

Recession   0 = none, 1 = mild, 2 = moderate, 3 = severe

Entry of air   0 = normal, 1 = decreased, 3 = markedly decreased

<2 mild, 3–5 moderate, 6+ severe.

Hypoxia and tiring are late signs.

Consider safe for discharge

Well with no significant respiratory distress at rest or after ED play

Normal observations

Playing normally and no agitation

Suitable home environment

Carers no longer concerned

Eating and drinking adequately

No fever >38°C while in ED

Written advice card and safety net advice given

Croup management approach

Ensure correct diagnosis and have considered all other causes of stridor in children.

Avoid distressing child, leave in comfortable position with carer.

Do not insert tongue depressor, take bloods or X-ray.

Assess for severity.

Steroids – Dexamethasone 0.15 mg/kg PO or nebulized 2 mg budesonide.

Observe.

If features of severe/deterioration

Nebulized adrenaline 0.5 mL/kg 1:1000 (max 5 mL).

100% oxygen as tolerated. Ensure adequate hydration.

Call senior paediatrician, senior ENT, PICU/ICU.

Consider intubation if evidence of impending respiratory failure, worsening hypoxia, respiratory rate >60 despite treatment, or falling respiratory rate without improvement, normal or rising CO_2, exhaustion. (Is it definitely croup?)

SAFEGUARDING

BRUISING IN CHILDREN

Features of a bruise to be considered as potentially resulting from maltreatment

Shape of a hand, ligature, stick, tooth marks, grip or implement imprint

Clear demarcation

Bruising or petechiae that are not explained by a medical condition (e.g. coagulopathy)

Bruising in non-ambulant child (e.g. child that does not roll yet or child with cerebral palsy who cannot move independently)

Multiple bruises

Multiple of similar shapes and sizes

In clusters

Away from bony prominences

Face, back, abdominal, arm, buttock, ear and hand bruises

On the neck that look like attempted strangulation

On the ankles and wrists that look like ligature marks

CONCERNING BURNS

Symmetrical hands or feet distribution

Circumferential distribution on limb

Absence of splash marks

Sparing in flexion creases

Area not expected to be in contact with hot object (back of hand, sole of feet, back, buttocks)

Cigarette shaped

NOTES:

Other concerning history features:

History inadequate, vague or inconsistent or no suitable explanation given

History not appropriate for child's age

Unwitnessed injury

Delayed presentation beyond what a 'reasonable' parent would do

Injury in under one year

Previous similar injuries/multiple attendances

Concerns about child's demeanour/parent-child interaction

READING

CEM clinical standards for emergency departments Feb 2013 – safeguarding children. Available from: http://www.collemergencymed.ac.uk/Shop-Floor/Clinical%20 Standards/default.asp

NICE guidelines (CG89). When to expect child maltreatment. March 2013.

PARENTAL RESPONSIBILITY UK

A mother automatically has parental responsibility (PR) for her child from birth.

A father has parental responsibility if he:

> is married to the child's mother at time of birth
>
> is listed on the birth certificate (from Dec 2003 England and Wales, Apr 2002 Northern Ireland, May 2006 Scotland)
>
> has jointly adopted a child
>
> has entered into a PR agreement with the mother
>
> has been issued a PR order from a court

Local authorities have PR if the child is subject to a care order.

Adoptive parents who jointly adopt a child have PR.

Parents do not lose PR if they divorce.

A guardian who will have PR can be appointed by a court.

READING

BMA Ethics Department – Parental Responsibility. 2008.

GMC 0–18 Years: Guidance for all Doctors. Appendix 2. 2007.

CALDICOTT PRINCIPLES

Caldicott principles when handling confidential patient data

Justify the purpose(s) for using patient data

Don't use patient-identifiable information unless it is absolutely necessary

Use the minimum necessary patient-identifiable information

Access to patient-identifiable information should be on a strict need-to-know basis

Everyone should be aware of their responsibilities to maintain confidentiality

Understand and comply with the law, in particular the Data Protection Act

The duty to share information can be as important as the duty to protect patient confidentiality

NOTES:

A Caldicott Guardian is a senior NHS person who is responsible for ensuring that his or her organization adheres to the Caldicott principles and ensures patient data is kept secure. It is now a requirement for every NHS organization to have a Caldicott guardian.

READING

The *Caldicott Report*. 1997.

Information: To share or not to share? *The Information Governance Review*. 2013.

SPINAL

AUTONOMIC DYSREFLEXIA

Phenomenon occurs in patients with spinal injuries at or above T6. An irritating stimulus occurring below the level of injury causes uncontrolled sympathetic activity, in particular severe hypertension. Can be life threatening, including cerebral haemorrhage.

Symptoms (only one or several symptoms may be present)

Headache pounding	Anxiety
Feeling of doom	Nasal stuffiness
Nausea	Dilated pupils
Sweating above cord lesion level	Chest tightness
Bradycardia	Flushing/blotching above cord lesion level
Hypertension	Penile erection
Goose bumps above or below cord lesion level	Cardiac arrhythmias
Vision blur or spots	Contraction of bladder and bowel

Precipitants include

Bladder	Over-distension, blocked catheter/tubing/full drainage bag, UTI, stones (bladder problems are the most common precipitants)
Bowel	Constipation, digital evacuation, rectal examination, haemorrhoids, appendicitis
Skin	Pressure sores, abrasions, abscesses, fractures, ingrown toe nails, burns, blisters
Other	Tight clothes/shoes, pregnancy, labour, sexual activity, menstruation, DVT

Treatment approach

Keep in sitting position.

Measure BP.

Thoroughly examine for and remove/treat precipitant. Start with assessing catheter patency. Perform PR with anaesthetic gel.

Sublingual nifedipine 10 mg or GTN.

Diazepam for spasms/fits.

Paracetamol/codeine for analgesia (avoid NSAIDs).

Discuss with local spinal injury unit.

NOTES:

Tetraplegic patients can be relatively hypotensive as their norm, e.g. systolic of 90. A rise of 20–40 mm Hg can be significant.

BACK PAIN RED FLAGS

Thoracic pain

Onset less than 20 yrs or
over 55 yrs of age

Bowel or bladder incontinence/
retention

Reduced anal tone

Neurological deficit/signs

Fever or recent treatment for sepsis

Saddle anaesthesia

Previous malignancy

Abdominal aortic aneurysm

Weight loss (unexplained)

Progressive pain not relieved by rest

Immunosuppressed

Intravenous drug use

HIV

Longstanding steroid use

Structural spinal abnormality

Recent trauma

Night pain

NOTES:

Surface anatomy landmarks:

C7	lowest prominent C spine process
T3	spinous process of scapula
T7	inferior tip of scapula
L4	iliac crests
Tip coccyx	ischeal tuberosities

Deep tendon reflexes:

Biceps C5, C6
Supinator C5, C6
Triceps C7, C8
Knee, L3, L4
Ankle S1

READING

NICE guidelines (CG88). Low back pain. May 2009.

SPINAL SYNDROMES

Anterior cord syndrome

Motor paralysis, pain and temperature loss. Vibration, proprioception intact.

Anterior cord infarction due to vascular insufficiency from anterior spinal artery.

Brown-Sequard syndrome

Ipsilateral motor paralysis and loss of proprioception and vibration.
Contralateral loss of temperature and pain.
Hemisection of cord, most commonly due to penetrating trauma.

Central cord syndrome

Motor deficit worse in upper limbs than lower. Varying sensory deficit.
Neck hyperextension injuries.

Cauda equine syndrome

Unilateral or bilateral perineal (saddle) sensory changes with motor and sensory deficits in legs. Bladder, bowel and sexual dysfunction. Lower back pain.

Compression of nerve roots below the conus medullaris.

READING

Guideline on the management of alert, adult patients with potential cervical spine injury in the Emergency Department. CEM 2010.

NICE guidelines (CG56). Selection of adults and children for imaging of the cervical spine. Head injury. September 2007.

Stiell IG et al. Implementation of the Canadian C-Spine Rule. Prospective 12 centre cluster randomised trial. *BMJ*. 2009;339:b4146.

TOXICOLOGY

**What are the contraindications for the
use of activated charcoal?
What are the indications for multidose activated charcoal?**

ACTIVATED CHARCOAL

A porous form of carbon that has a large surface area.

Contraindications and cautions

Risk of pulmonary aspiration (causes severe inhalation injury)
Bowel obstruction (cannot ultimately be excreted)
Ingestion of an acid, an alkali or a petroleum product (impedes ability to
physically see GI tract damage during endoscopy)
Unpalatable and causes vomiting
Substances not bound to charcoal

MULTIPLE-DOSE ACTIVATED CHARCOAL

Repeated doses of charcoal at 4-hour intervals, up to a total of four doses, have
been shown to increase elimination for a small number of drugs (including car-
bamazepine, digoxin, theophylline).

NOTES:

Activated charcoal binds toxin to prevent stomach and intestinal absorption.
Toxins therefore stay within the GI tract and are removed in stools. Interrupts
enterohepatic and enteroenteric circulation of some drugs/toxins and their
metabolites.
Effect decreases with time post ingestion – therefore is used within one hour of
ingestion.
Can be given orally or via NG tube.
Dose adults 50 g, children 1 g/kg (can mix with fruit juice to disguise taste).

READING

http://www.toxbase.org

ACCIDENTAL INJECTION OF EPIPEN (ADRENALINE) INTO THUMB/FINGER

Results in digit pain, paraesthesia, pallor and coolness due to vasoconstriction, occasionally with potential for tissue ischaemia.

Minimal symptoms – Place affected digit into bowl of warm water, observe and arrange follow-up at 24 and 48 hr.

Significant features – Local injection of phentolamine +/– local injection of lignocaine.

NOTES:

Differential diagnosis of angioedema: allergic, hereditary, ACE inhibitors, idiopathic.

Potential anaphylaxis triggers include

Stings (wasp, bee)
Food (nuts, eggs)
Drugs (antibiotics, anaesthetics, vaccines)
Contrast media
Latex

Mast cell tryptase levels

Useful for follow-up of suspected anaphylactic reactions.
Send samples after resuscitation has started, at 1–2 hr, at 24 hr/in OPD clinic.

READING

Emergency treatment of anaphylactic reactions. Resuscitation council (UK) update 2012. Available from: http://www.resus.org.uk/pages/reaction.pdf (includes drugs and drug doses).

NICE guidelines (CG134). Anaphylaxis: assessment to confirm an anaphylactic episode and the decision to refer after emergency treatment for a suspected anaphylactic episode. December 2011.

WERNICKE KORSAKOFF

Wernicke encephalopathy

Acute, reversible triad of acute confusion, ataxia, and ophthalmoplegia due to thiamine deficiency.

Causes
> Chronic alcohol excess
> Malnutrition
> Malignancy
> Eating disorders
> Hyperemesis gravidarum
> HIV
> Dialysis

Investigations (to also exclude other differential diagnoses)
> Blood test – FBC, UE, LFT, glucose, arterial blood gas, cholesterol, thiamine levels
> LP
> CT/MRI brain

Management – IV thiamine as Pabrinex (two pairs of vials 1 and 2 diluted in 100 mL of crystalloid IV over 30 min acutely in the ED and continued tds for two days if admitted)

Korsakoff syndrome

Irreversible confabulation, retrograde amnesia and memory loss due to thiamine deficiency

NOTES:

Patients with a history of chronic alcohol ingestion or other risk factors for thiamine deficiency who receive IV dextrose (e.g. to treat hypoglycaemia) should also immediately receive IV Pabrinex.

READING

NICE guidelines (CG100). Alcohol-use disorders: Diagnosis and clinical management of alcohol-related physical complications. June 2010.

NICE guidelines (CG115). Alcohol-use disorders: Diagnosis, assessment and management of harmful drinking and alcohol dependence. February 2011.

METHAEMOGLOBINAEMIA

Methaemoglobinaemia results from elevated levels of methaemoglobin in the blood (normal levels <1%). The haemoglobin molecule ferrous (Fe^{2+}), which is oxygen carrying, is oxidized to the ferric form (Fe^{3+}), which reduces oxygen release to tissues.

Presentation

Classical presentation
> Chocolate brown-coloured blood
> Cyanosis unresponsive to oxygenation
> pO_2 is normal but measured oxygen saturations are low

Symptoms relate to concentration:
> 10–30% blue-grey discolouration, lethargy, headaches
> >50% seizures, reduced GCS, respiratory depression, arrhythmias
> >70% potentially fatal

Patients with pre-existing cardiac and respiratory disease, sepsis or sickle cell are likely to experience more significant symptoms at lower levels.

Treatment approach

High flow oxygen

Methylene blue (methylthioninium). Refer to toxbase and discuss with national poisons information service. Reduces ferric back to normal ferrous iron.

Remove cause/prevent further absorption

Causes

Congenital (autosomal recessive)

Acquired, including poppers (nitrites), nitrates, trimethoprim, local anaesthetics (prilocaine, lignocaine)

READING

http://www.toxbase.org

ORGANOPHOSPHATE POISONING

Presentation

Agitation	Bradycardia and tachyarrhythmias
Bronchial hypersecretion	Confusion
Diarrhoea	Lacrimation
Hypotension	Miosis
Muscle fasciculations	Respiratory failure
Rhinorrhoea	Salivation
Sweating	Urinary retention
Weakness/exhaustion	

Organophosphates are found in pesticides and nerve gases. They inhibit acetylcholinesterase, resulting in the lack of degradation of acetylcholine causing excessive muscarinic and nicotinic receptor stimulation in the ANS and CNS. Toxicity can result from inhalation, ingestion, skin or eye exposure, with symptoms occurring at exposure or up to 12 hours later. Toxicity is a clinical diagnosis based on the presenting toxidrome. Cholinesterase levels can be measured in the blood (send EDTA sample). Avoid self-contamination with PPE and decontamination. Antidotes are atropine (antimuscarinic) and pralidoxime (reactivates AChE by binding to organophosphates).

NOTES:
Other antidotes:

Beta blockers	Glucagon
Cyanide	Dicobalt edentate, sodium thiosulphate, hydroxocobalamin
Ethylene glycol	Fomepizole, alcohol
Extrapyramidal side effects	Procyclidine
Hydrofluoric acid	Calcium gluconate gel
Iron	Desferrioxamine
Methaemoglobinaemia	Methylene blue
Opiates	Naloxone
Paracetamol	N-acetylcysteine

READING

http://www.toxbase.org includes drug doses of antidotes.

ANION GAP

Calculating the anion gap can help differentiate the cause of a metabolic acidosis.

Formula:

$$(Na^+ + K^+) - (Cl^- + HCO_3^-)$$

Normal range = 8–12

High anion gap metabolic acidosis causes (mnemonic MUD PILES)

Methanol
Uraemia
DKA
Paraldehyde poisoning
Iron poisoning
Lactic acidosis
Ethylene glycol poisoning
Salicylate poisoning

Normal anion gap metabolic acidosis causes (mnemonic FUSED CAR)

Fistulae
Uretogastric conduits
Saline administration
Endocrine – Addison, hyperparathyroidism
Diarrhoea
Carbonic anhydrase inhibitors
Ammonium chloride
Renal tubular acidosis

Low anion gap metabolic acidosis causes

Hyperparaproteinaemia
Hypoalbuminaemia

OSMOLAR GAP

$$\text{Calculated osmolality} = 2 \times (Na) + \text{urea} + \text{glucose}$$
Normal range 285–295 mOsm/kg
$$\text{Osmolar gap} = (\text{measured osmolality}) - (\text{calculated osmolality})$$
Normal range less than 10

Causes of high osmolar gap

Methanol
Ethylene glycol
Ethanol
Mannitol
Sorbitol
Acetone
DKA
Propylene glycol (found in IV lorazepam)
Alcoholic ketoacidosis
Myeloma (increased plasma proteins)
Hyperlipidaemia

INHALATION INJURY

Associated clinical features

Facial, neck or lip burns
Breathlessness
Carbonaceous sputum
Wheezing
Blistering/oedema of mouth
Cough
Soot visible mouth or nose
Stridor
Singed facial/forehead hair
Hoarse voice
Nausea/vomiting
Hypoxia
Dizziness
Confusion
Headache
Bronchoscopy or laryngeal evidence of contamination

NOTES:

Smoke inhalation causes a combination of a thermal injury, systemic toxicity (e.g. carbon monoxide and hydrogen cyanide poisoning) and lung injury from particle deposits and pulmonary irritants. Consider also associated trauma (falls from height/stairs escaping a blast) and hypothermia (extended cold water first aid). Significant inhalation injuries can be relatively asymptomatic initially, with clinical deterioration at 12 to 24 hrs+. A history of loss of consciousness or entrapment at the scene is significant. Assess for corneal burns with fluorescein and measure carboxyhaemoglobin levels.

INDICATIONS FOR STARTING RENAL REPLACEMENT THERAPY

Hyperkalaemia
Potassium persistently >6.5
Severe acidaemia pH<7.1
Significant uraemia >30 mmol/L
Uraemia complications – pericarditis, myopathy, encephalopathy, neuropathy
Oliguria <200 mL in 12 hours
Significant hyperthermia
Significant hypothermia
Significant volume overload
Persistent severe hypercalcaemia >4.5
Persistent severe hypermagnesaemia
Persistent severe acute hyponatraemia <115 or hypernatraemia >160
Drug overdose, including lithium, aminoglycosides, salicylates, methanol

NOTES:

Not all drugs are removed by haemodialysis.

LOCAL ANAESTHETIC (LA) TOXICITY

Local anaesthetic calculation examples

Maximum dose of 1% lignocaine for a seven-year-old

> Maximum safe dose lignocaine is 3 mg/kg, seven-year-old weight 22 kg, therefore = 66 mg
>
> 1% lignocaine solution contains 10 mg/mL, therefore maximum volume is 6.6 mL

Maximum dose of 0.5% bupivicaine for a five-year-old

> Max safe dose bupivicaine is 2 mg/kg, five-year-old weight 18 kg, therefore = 36 mg
>
> 0.5% bupivicaine solution contains 5 mg/mL, therefore maximum volume is 7.2 mL

Volumes calculated are the maximum safe volume, not the volume aiming to be used.

Presentation of LA toxicity

Neurological symptoms (CNS excitation followed by CNS depression) then cardiovascular symptoms

> Perioral and tongue paraesthesia, light-headedness, visual disturbances, headaches, restlessness
>
> Dysarthria, tinnitus, metallic taste
>
> Muscle twitching, drowsiness
>
> Seizures, reduced GCS
>
> Respiratory arrest
>
> Tachycardia, hypertension then hypotension
>
> Cardiovascular depression and arrhythmias

NOTES:

LA toxicity occurs following an excessive dose or accidental intravascular administration.

Early features can be subtle in children or sedated patients, with first symptom as CVS collapse. Large bolus injections can cause simultaneous CNS and CVS features. Toxicity can also occur late at 10–25 mins post injection.

Drug concentration is expressed as a percentage (e.g. bupivacaine 0.25%, lignocaine 1%).

Percentage is measured in grams per 100 mL (i.e. 1% is 1 g/100 mL).

Therefore 1 mL of 1% lignocaine contains 10 mg of lignocaine.

READING

Association of Anaesthetists of Great Britain and Ireland. Management of severe local anaesthetic toxicity. 2010. Available from: http://www.aagbi.org

INDEX